28-DAY
FAST
START
DAY-BY-DAY

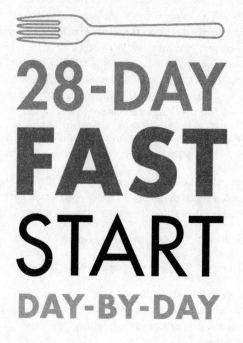

28-DAY
FAST
START
DAY-BY-DAY

THE ULTIMATE GUIDE TO STARTING
(OR RESTARTING) YOUR INTERMITTENT FASTING
LIFESTYLE SO IT STICKS

GIN STEPHENS

ST. MARTIN'S
GRIFFIN
NEW YORK

First published in the United States by St. Martin's Griffin, an imprint of St. Martin's Publishing Group

28-DAY FAST START DAY-BY-DAY. Copyright © 2023 by Gin Stephens. All rights reserved. Printed in the United States of America. For information, address St. Martin's Publishing Group, 120 Broadway, New York, NY 10271.

www.stmartins.com

Library of Congress Cataloging-in-Publication Data

Names: Stephens, Gin, author.
Title: 28-day fast start day-by-day: the ultimate guide to starting (or restarting) your intermittent fasting lifestyle so it sticks / Gin Stephens.
Other titles: Twenty-eight-day fast start day-by-day
Description: First edition. | New York: St. Martin's Griffin, 2023. | Includes index.
Identifiers: LCCN 2023031041 | ISBN 9781250824172 (trade paperback) | ISBN 9781250824189 (ebook)
Subjects: LCSH: Intermittent fasting. | Reducing diets. | Weight loss. | Natural foods.
Classification: LCC RM226 .S74 2023 | DDC 613.2/5—dc23/eng/20230817
LC record available at https://lccn.loc.gov/2023031041

Our books may be purchased in bulk for promotional, educational, or business use. Please contact your local bookseller or the Macmillan Corporate and Premium Sales Department at 1-800-221-7945, extension 5442, or by email at MacmillanSpecialMarkets@macmillan.com.

First Edition: 2023

10 9 8 7 6 5 4 3 2 1

CONTENTS

28-DAY
FAST
START
DAY-BY-DAY

WELCOME! START HERE

I'm so glad you picked up a copy of this book, or maybe a good friend or family member who is an intermittent faster gave you a copy to introduce you to intermittent fasting (which we call *IF*).

First, I want to explain what this book *is* and what it *isn't*.

My goal with this book is to take you by the hand and walk with you as you begin your journey down the IF path. As we go along together throughout the next month, I want to equip you with the tools you need so that IF sticks.

Here's what this book *is*:

As it says right in the title, it's your 28-Day FAST Start day-by-day guide to starting (or restarting) your IF lifestyle so it sticks.

What this book *isn't*: a complete guide to all-things IF. That's a different book: *Fast. Feast. Repeat.: The Comprehensive Guide to Delay, Don't Deny Intermittent Fasting.*

I want to be very clear:

The book you are holding is a companion to *Fast. Feast. Repeat.* If you could only get *one* book, that's the one you want. (Don't tell my publisher I said that.)

But you really need BOTH books. *And this is not just me selling you two books. I promise. You're going to save so much money on food and fancy coffee drinks this month that* *you could afford to buy thirty books with the money you'll save. Another benefit of IF! You're welcome. ;-)*

So, why do you need two books, when *Fast. Feast. Repeat.* has everything you need to begin and implement an intermittent fasting lifestyle successfully, and to tweak it till it's easy?

You could say that's *Fast. Feast. Repeat.'s* greatest strength: it's comprehensive.

But you could also say it's the book's greatest *weakness*.

What do I mean by that? It's so complete that it can be overwhelming.

I hear comments like this one all the time: "*I gave a copy of* Fast. Feast. Repeat. *to my sister and she says it's too long and she won't read it.*"

Or someone will read *Fast. Feast. Repeat.* cover to cover and then feel like their brain is so overflowing with information that they don't know what to do next.

Information overload.

And that is why this day-by-day guide was born. Not everyone is ready for ALL of the science found in *Fast. Feast. Repeat.* on day 1 of their journey.

"*Just tell me exactly what to do, Gin!*"

That's what you have here. For the next month, I'm going to guide you through each day. This book is consumable and designed for you to write in as you go. If it helps, think about it as your IF success journal. I was a teacher for twenty-eight years, so my expertise is curriculum design: I'm trained to present content and to make sure it sticks. And I'm using many of the strategies I learned as an effective teacher here in this book.

Every day, you'll begin the day by confirming your daily fasting plan and setting your intention by creating achievable goals. There will be a daily lesson from me designed to give you the knowledge and motivation you need to keep going (even when it gets hard). All but a few of these lessons are short and sweet on purpose so you don't get bogged down by too much information.

You'll also hear from a past *Intermittent Fasting Stories* podcast guest in a Daily Inspiration Spotlight. Along with reading an update, where they share what's been happening since their interview, you may want to find their podcast episode (on your favorite podcast app or at intermittentfastingstories.com) to hear their entire inspiring story. The Daily Inspiration Spotlights will provide even more inspiration to your day.

At the end of each day, you'll take a few minutes to reflect on how the day went, including both the fast *and* the feast. You'll identify what went well and what might have been a struggle. You'll also think about the next day, always looking ahead and planning for success.

But don't forget that while you work through this book for the next month, you're also going to need a copy of *Fast. Feast. Repeat.* as a reference. After a few of the daily lessons, I'll point you toward sections of *Fast. Feast. Repeat.* where you can go for more in-depth information about the daily topic. I'm calling them your "extra credit reading" assignments. Yep—I'm still a teacher at heart. Since it's extra credit, I know that you might not have time to get to each of them, but they are there for you when you want or need more information.

If you don't yet have a copy of *Fast. Feast. Repeat.*, go ahead and order it now. You won't be sorry—it's going to be an integral part of your long-term success. Also, all the scientific research and references are contained in *Fast. Feast.*

Repeat., as are the next steps that you'll need after your FAST Start is over.

But for now: it's most important that you stick with me *here* in this day-by-day guide and concentrate on one thing only: building up your fasting muscle and establishing IF as a habit. When you take it day by day, you won't be overwhelmed, and you'll set yourself up for long-term success.

Are you excited? Let's do this!

WHAT IS "INTERMITTENT FASTING"?

If you are new to IF, you may wonder: What exactly is intermittent fasting? Even if you eat three meals a day plus snacks like most people in our modern society, you are somewhat of a faster, whether you realize it or not. We all fast while we sleep, and we wake up every morning in a fasted state. Most intermittent fasters simply extend that fasted state throughout the day rather than eating a traditional breakfast in the morning. Just like everyone else, we break-fast, but it may be when most people are having their lunch or dinner. *Breakfast* literally means "break the fast." We all do it, just at different times of the day. For me, break-fast, which I usually eat in the late afternoon or early evening, really is the most important meal of the day!

For intermittent fasters, there's a period of the day when we intentionally fast, sticking to clean-fast-approved beverages only (plain water, black coffee, plain tea, and unflavored sparkling water)—and there's a period of the day when we eat, which is called our *eating window*. I'll help you choose your preferred eating window approach for the FAST Start before you begin, so keep reading.

It's important to understand that IF is a flexible lifestyle that doesn't have to be exactly the same from day to day, but the most common eating windows vary between one and eight hours a day.

To illustrate how this looks, let's say someone follows an intermittent fasting lifestyle with a four-hour daily eating window. Since a day has twenty-four hours, twenty hours of each day (including the time you are asleep) would be spent fasting, and all your eating for the day would take place during the consecutive four-hour eating window that you choose. We would call that approach 20:4, representing twenty hours of fasting and a four-hour eating window. Most people who use the daily eating window approach end up with anything between 16:8 (sixteen hours of fasting and an eight-hour eating window) and 23:1 (a twenty-three-hour fast and a one-hour eating window). Because it's a flexible lifestyle, your eating window can vary from day to day, based on your schedule and even your varying appetite.

Here's how this might look as a day in my life. Every morning, I wake up and start the day with black coffee. After my coffee, I switch over to water and unflavored sparkling water until I am ready to eat. I usually open my eating window at some point between 2:00 and 5:00 p.m. with a snack of some type. A couple of hours later, I prepare dinner for my husband and me, and we eat together. After dinner, I will often have a dessert of some type, or just a little something sweet to close my window. Overall, my eating window lasts for somewhere between two and six hours most days.

The daily eating window approach isn't the only way to live an intermittent fasting lifestyle, and there are other options that involve longer fasts of up to thirty-six to forty-two hours. These are based on the concept of alternate daily fasting (ADF), which is a well-researched practice. ADF isn't something you're going to implement during your FAST Start, so I won't explain it here. It's a tool that is described fully within *Fast. Feast. Repeat.*, and something you can consider for later in your IF journey.

You may be wondering:

Is intermittent fasting extreme or dangerous?

For people who have never heard of intermittent fasting or who don't understand the many health benefits that come along with the IF lifestyle (which I will cover on day 4), this type of schedule may seem bizarre or even possibly dangerous. What?!?!?! You go most of the day without eating? Every *day*? You might even fast for thirty-six hours? Don't you have headaches? Don't you collapse from lack of food? How do you have energy to do day-to-day tasks?

Many intermittent fasters have gotten the speeches from well-meaning friends and family members:

"Of course you're losing weight, you're starving yourself!"
"Everyone knows that breakfast is the most important meal of the day! You need energy to start your day."

Neither of those statements is true, even though we have probably all heard them. You aren't starving yourself, and you won't collapse without breakfast. Let's dig into each of them:

Are we starving ourselves? Absolutely not. My comprehensive book is called *Fast. **Feast**. Repeat.* after all, not *Fast. **Eat a little tiny diet meal**. Repeat.*

When I eat, I eat well, and that's true for most IFers. I choose foods that make me feel great, and I eat until I am satisfied. Back in my low-calorie diet days, whenever I wanted to lose a few pounds, I would restrict my calories throughout the day to about 1,200 (because that's what "they" said I should do), and *that* felt like I was starving myself. I'll explain more about how IF is different from a low-calorie diet on day 3.

What about breakfast? Do we need breakfast first thing in the morning to fuel our bodies? The surprising answer to that question is no. If you have ever been hangry, you know the feeling. You need to eat NOW. Many people imagine that is what IF feels like. While it may feel like that over the brief adjustment period, once we are adapted, *hangry* goes away. The key is that we are well fueled during the fast . . . by our fat stores, which exist for that very purpose. One of the most common things we hear from new IFers is that they can't believe how great they feel during the fast. Most of us are a lot less hungry while fasting than back in our low-calorie or frequent-small-meal days. The difference is astounding. Instead of getting worse over time, like most low-calorie diets, IF gets better and better as we adjust. More about this on days 9 and 16.

For now, what you need to remember is this: as we progress through the 28-Day FAST Start Day by Day, I'll teach you everything you need to know about intermittent fasting so that you understand the basics and have the tools you need to set a firm IF foundation . . . and ensure that your IF lifestyle *sticks*.

WHY DO IFERS QUIT? AND HOW TO KEEP IT FROM HAPPENING TO *YOU*

Maybe you have never heard of IF before today, and you think it sounds too good to be true. Good news! It *isn't* too good to be true, as you will learn for yourself over time. The intermittent fasting lifestyle has changed thousands (if not millions) of lives, and yours is about to be one of them.

Or maybe you've dabbled with IF in the past but couldn't make it stick. The book you are holding is designed to equip you with all the tools you need to make sure it sticks this time. There are a few common mistakes you may have made in the past that I'm going to help you identify. And once you identify what was holding you back, you'll be prepared for success.

It's even possible that you lived as an IFer for a significant period of time, but for whatever reason, you have wandered off the path and are looking for your way back to the lifestyle that you *know* is right for you. The next month is designed to ease you back into IF. Think of it as your *fresh* start.

You may be reading this and asking:

If IF is so great, why would anyone quit?

That's a great question, and I am glad you asked. I've had amazing success with IF, but for years I fit into the category of "couldn't make it stick." You see, I was an IF dabbler. In my heart of hearts, I had the feeling that intermittent fasting was the answer. Unfortunately, however, I didn't have the tools that I needed to make IF into a *lifestyle*.

I treated IF as if it were another diet. I would start, last a few days, and then get discouraged for whatever reason:

» **Results were neither quick nor dramatic.** I had unrealistic expectations. *(Blame the tabloids at the checkout counter of the grocery store that tell you you'll lose ____ pounds by ____. You won't, because that is not how the body works. But it makes you think you **should** be able to do it. When you don't, you blame yourself, of course, when really it was the unrealistic expectations that failed you.)*

» **It was *hard*.** I didn't understand the adjustment period, or what needed to go on within my body during the adaptation process. So, as soon as it felt hard, I quit.

» **Food soothed me in times of stress.** I was an elementary school teacher, a mom of two school-aged boys, a wife, and I also had a second (and third, and fourth) job teaching adults in two online universities and our school district's gifted teacher endorsement program. When I wasn't busy with family or work, I turned to food. Food was always there, and it didn't talk back.

Is it any wonder that I kept quitting?

I'm not going to let that happen to you. Not this time.

I've been around the intermittent fasting world since 2009, first as a *dabbler* (2009–2014) and then as a *newly determined IFer* who felt like this was her final shot (2014–2015). Starting in 2015, I transformed into an *excited IFer* who had finally reached her goal weight (after years of failed diets), and I started my first IF support group on Facebook. That allowed me to mentor hundreds of thousands of IFers from around the world, and inspired me to write my first book (*Delay, Don't Deny*, in 2016) and become a podcaster in 2017.

Since that happened, I have gone on to reach millions of listeners and readers through my books and podcasts and to write the *New York Times* bestseller *Fast. Feast. Repeat.*, and I am grateful to have the opportunity to continue to mentor intermittent fasters through my online support community. We are no longer on Facebook these days, and you can find us by going to ginstephens.com/community.

In my IF evolution, I am now an *experienced IFer*. As of the writing of this book, I have gone through *nine* holiday seasons as an intermittent faster. Nine summers, vacations and all. This is the first time in my adult life that I have stuck to something for this long.

And I know this:

I will never stop living the intermittent fasting lifestyle.

My experience, plus the experience of thousands of other successful IFers, illustrates that IF is a lifestyle that works long term.

Just ask Dr. Mark Mattson, who I interviewed for episode 204 of my podcast, *Intermittent Fasting Stories*. He is one of the world's leading experts on intermittent fasting, and he has been living the IF lifestyle since the 1980s. Dr. Mattson is the former chief of the Laboratory of Neurosciences at the National Institute on Aging, and he is best known for cutting-edge neurological research during his time at Johns Hopkins University. When someone with that level of scientific expertise tells me that he chooses to live the intermittent fasting lifestyle because he is sold on the profound health benefits, I listen.

And he's not the only researcher who is sold on the health benefits of IF. Dr. Gil Blander appeared on episode 96 of the *Intermittent Fasting Stories* podcast. He received his Ph.D. from MIT with a focus on aging research, and he is considered to be an expert in the area of longevity. As of my interview with him in 2020, he had been living the IF lifestyle for eight years, and he told me: "The best intervention we have available for us today to live longer is IF. It is natural and simple. It's not easy for the first couple of weeks. But once it becomes a routine, then it's easy." (He's right, by the way. Even though it might not be easy on day 1, once you are fully adapted, it becomes something you simply *do*.)

Besides talking to scientists and experts who choose to live the IF lifestyle, I have interviewed hundreds of IF-ers from the real world who are just like you and me. They are like your neighbor, your mom, your friend, your son or daughter . . . real-life people who have made the intermittent fasting lifestyle work for them long term.

It is the greatest joy of my life to talk to successful intermittent fasters and hear how IF has transformed them and their lives in ways they never expected.

Even so, sometimes I talk to people who have struggled

to make IF work for them. Not every story begins as a success story. Mine didn't.

You're probably not surprised (especially if you've ever listened to me on podcasts) that I love to talk to people about IF. And that includes perfect strangers. Just imagine how many grocery store checkout lane conversations or random encounters I have had that ended up turning to IF. Oops. What can I say? I'm passionate about the topic. You don't lose eighty pounds and keep it off and not want to shout it from the mountaintops.

In the early years of my IF journey, it was common for people to have never heard of IF. Frankly, many of them thought it sounded crazy. "Thank you, Crazy Grocery Store Lady. Please allow me to check out with my groceries now."

But somewhere around 2019, the tide began to shift. Now, when I bring up IF with a stranger, it seems they all know someone who has had great success with it.

These days, it's very common that the person I'm talking to even tried it themselves at some point. For those who have tried it, the conversation usually goes something like this:

STRANGER: *I tried it, and it didn't work for me.*
ME: *Tell me about that. What were you drinking during the fast?*

BOOM!
That's when they tell me about the energy drinks, or the coffee with cream, or the flavored sparkling water, or the herbal tea, or the _____—you can fill in the blank with any number of beverages that break a fast, making it

much harder to get through the day. More about why in the next chapter, where I will give you the basics of what I call the *clean fast*. Trust me when I tell you that the clean fast changes everything.

Sometimes, however, the person I'm talking to *did* fast clean. Maybe they only drank plain water, and they stuck to black coffee.

When someone who was fasting clean tells me that IF "didn't work for them," my next question is usually:

How long did you give it, and how did you determine it wasn't working for you?

Every time, the answer is some sort of combination of only giving it a couple of weeks at the most, and they were usually using the lack of dramatic scale movement to determine that IF "wasn't working."

If you've tried IF in the past and quit, I bet you either weren't fasting clean, or you didn't give it long enough.

But that doesn't apply to someone who lived the IF lifestyle successfully for a time, fasted clean, had great results, and then quit. Why does that happen? Did that happen to *you*, by any chance? There can be many reasons you stopped fasting:

» **You followed bad advice**—There's a lot of conflicting information out there, and if you go down every path, you can lose your way. Instead, keep it simple: fast clean, and learn to listen to your own body and to trust yourself.

» **Life got in the way**—Maybe a vacation happened and you never went back to intermittent fasting, or a stressful period of time caused you to stop fasting. Before you knew it, you were not fasting at all.

» **Diet brain took over**—Maybe your friend started a new diet plan and was losing weight more quickly than you were, so you decided fasting wasn't "working" and you jumped ship to this other plan.

» **You began to question fasting in general**—Maybe you saw a blog post or news article that made you question either the safety or efficacy of IF. *(As an example, in late 2022, a bunch of articles came out that claimed certain dangers associated with IF, but when I looked into the study the articles were based on, I realized **it wasn't a fasting study** . . . by the way, this is actually a common tactic in what passes for health journalism these days—sensational headlines that don't reflect what the study actually found or even what it actually studied. Always go to the source rather than trusting the headlines.)*

» **Naysayers got into your head**—Sadly, this is very common. Someone you know (or even someone you love) plants a seed or disparages fasting, or makes you feel silly or even guilty about your choices. So, you quit.

If you quit, don't let that stop you from trying again. Think about a toddler who is learning to walk. That toddler doesn't fall down once and say, "Welp. Looks like walking isn't for me." No. That toddler gets up and tries again, as many times as it takes.

Have you heard the Japanese proverb:

Fall down seven times, get up eight.

If this is your first time as an IFer, the tools in this book will give you a great foundation to ensure you get up each time you fall down. If you've tried IF in the past, maybe you already know where you went wrong, and you're ready to get it *right* this time.

Either way, I hope you're excited, because this time, you are *not going to quit.*

Write it down:

I am not going to quit.

And sign your name to it. Date it. Make that promise to yourself today.

WHAT IS THE "CLEAN FAST"? THE BASICS

The clean fast is the one nonnegotiable rule that I will never waver on, and you shouldn't, either: when you fast, fast clean. Otherwise, you are not really fasting.

The clean fast is so important that I devoted *two* chapters of *Fast. Feast. Repeat.* to the topic. In chapter 4, "The Magic Is in the Clean Fast! Learn *Why* We Fast Clean," I explain the rationale behind the clean fast, with all the scientific explanations as to why it matters and why we care. In chapter 5, "Keep It Clean! Learn *How* We Fast Clean," I share all the details of what it means to fast clean, followed by ten pages of stories from forty-three IFers who share how the clean fast was instrumental in their success.

You need to read both of those chapters, because understanding *why* is a lot more powerful than simply hearing me tell you what to do. When you understand why, you'll never want to sacrifice the clean fast, and you'll prize that time of your day even more, recognizing how powerful it truly is.

So, your homework assignment is to read the clean fast chapters of *Fast. Feast. Repeat.* at some point in the near future to fully comprehend the *why* and the *how*.

For now, use this diagram to understand the clean fast.

WHAT IS A "CLEAN FAST"?		
YES!	MAYBE . . .	NO!
• Water (unflavored) • Black coffee (unflavored) • Any plain tea brewed from actual dried leaves only (black tea, green tea, etc., unflavored varieties only, loose or in tea bags) • Mineral water, club soda, sparkling water, or seltzer water (unflavored) • Minerals/electrolytes/salt (with no additives or flavors) • Medications as prescribed by your health care provider	*We call this the "gray area":* • Peppermint essential oil for breath freshening only, NOT for water-enhancing *(select food-grade and use sparingly)* • Herbal tea with a bitter flavor profile • Vitamins and supplements *(There is no easy answer for all vitamins and supplements. Any that are clearly food-like or listed in the "No" column should be taken within your eating window.)*	• Food • Flavored water • Flavored coffee • Fruity, sweet, or matcha teas • Diet sodas • Natural or artificial sweeteners • Gum or mints • Food-like flavors of any type *(fruit juices, fruit flavors, etc.)* • Bone broth, broth, or bouillon • Fat, including coconut oil, MCT oil, butter, etc. • Cream, creamers, milk, or milk substitutes *(of any amount or type)* • Supplements such as collagen, pre-workouts, BCAAs, exogenous ketones, etc.

Whenever you aren't sure if something is okay for the clean fast, take a look at the ingredients and compare them against this chart. If the item only contains ingredients from the "Yes" column, it's fine. If it has ingredients from the "No" column, it doesn't work. And, if it is something in the gray area, it may or may not work for you.

IMPORTANT: Don't experiment with anything from the gray area until after you complete the 28-Day FAST Start. At that point, you should know how your body feels during the clean fast. If you then experiment with a gray area item and you find it makes you hungry or shaky/nauseous within about an hour (or sooner), that is a clear signal that it doesn't work well for you during the fast. If the item is okay for you, you probably won't notice any difference in hunger or energy levels. You'll feel the same as you did when fasting clean. If that happens, congratulations! That item is probably fine for you. **By the way: This is never an excuse for trying anything from the "No" list. The *"does it make me hungry/shaky"* test isn't foolproof, and remember that you don't want to risk breaking your fast. Everything on the "No" list is *always* a no, for reasons that are fully explained in *Fast. Feast. Repeat.***

CHOOSE YOUR FAST START APPROACH

Much of this chapter is taken directly from *Fast. Feast. Repeat.*, and I'm including it here because I know you might not have had time to get a copy yet.

Before you begin your FAST Start, it's important to understand its purpose and choose your approach. This chapter will help you do that.

In the FAST Start, you will:

F = Fast Clean
A = Adapt
S = Settle In
T = Tweak

These are the four cornerstones of the FAST Start:

F=Fast Clean	This is not negotiable. Every minute you are fasting, follow the guidelines for the clean fast. During the first twenty-eight days, stick to items from the "yes" column only, and don't experiment with any of the items that are in the gray area.

A=Adapt	You will ignite your fat-burning superpower, and your body will physically adapt, learning how to tap into your fat stores over time.
S=Settle In	For each of the four weeks, you will settle in to a predictable fasting routine. Embrace the changes that you experience along the way (even the challenging ones!) and take note of how you feel as the weeks progress.
T=Tweak	While I will suggest an overall fasting routine for each week based on your personality type, feel free to change from one approach to another if you need to. Just because you decided you wanted to "rip off the Band-Aid" on day 1, that doesn't mean that you are stuck there! Head on down to the Easy Does It approach if you need to. It's okay! You can also tweak the time of day where your eating window falls from day to day to see what feels right to you.

Think of this first twenty-eight-day period as the time when you will lay the foundation for your intermittent fasting practice.

It's time to decide which of the three FAST Start plans is the best fit for you. Take this short quiz to figure it out. *(Or you can skip the quiz and go straight to the three plans and make your own choice. I have to admit: I am a sucker for a quiz, since I am a retired teacher. If you don't want to take a quiz, I forgive you. This is one more way that we are all different.)* This isn't a quiz that you can fail, which is good news.

1. **In the past, when you have started a new eating plan, which best describes you?**
   a. I like to read about the plan, spend several weeks gathering resources, and then ease my way in.

b. I make do with the foods I already have in my kitchen and gradually implement the suggestions over time.

c. I throw away all noncompliant foods and restock my kitchen completely to match my new plan. Let's go!

2. Which describes your decision-making process?

a. I like to take my time before coming to a decision, carefully weighing out all the pros and cons. I usually make some sort of list or ask for the opinion of others before deciding. I may have trouble making the decision.

b. I think about the options carefully and then feel confident in my decision.

c. I immediately know what my decision will be based on intuition and what feels right.

3. What has tripped you up the most on past diet or health plans?

a. I am easily overwhelmed when there are too many changes at once.

b. I don't always give myself enough time to adapt to the plan.

c. I am usually impatient and looking for quick results.

4. How do you face a difficult challenge?

a. If it seems too difficult, I may be discouraged and give up.

b. With time and effort, I usually accomplish what I set out to do.

c. Bring it on! I can do anything I set my mind to.

5. How is your health?

a. I have some health challenges, but my doctor said it is okay for me to start IF.

b. I am in pretty good health overall.

c. I am as healthy as a horse, thankyouverymuch.

TIME TO SCORE THE QUIZ!

Give yourself 0 points for every A, 2 points for every B, and 4 points for every C.

If you scored 0–4, you should start with the *Easy Does It* approach.

If you scored a 6, you should consider either the *Easy Does It* or *Steady Build* approach.

If you scored an 8–12, you should start with the *Steady Build* approach.

If you scored a 14, you should consider either the *Steady Build* or the *Rip Off the Band-Aid* approach.

If you scored a 16–20, you should start with the *Rip Off the Band-Aid* approach.

Feel free to ignore this quiz if you find it to be hokey, and choose whatever plan feels right to *you*. Remember: *you* are in charge at all times.

NOTE: Based on an informal survey of intermittent fasters, I found that 61 percent of IFers in my online community prefer an evening window while 25 percent prefer a midday eating window. For that reason, the FAST Start plan has been designed with an early-evening eating window as the goal. Feel free to adjust the window timing on any of these approaches as it feels right to you.

Let's dig into the three FAST Start approaches and see just how to implement each of them. Even though there are many tools in your intermittent fasting toolbox, the FAST Start will focus on the eating window approach to IF. After the first twenty-eight days are over, you will be free to pull out other tools and experiment with the other approaches. The other tools are fully explained in *Fast. Feast. Repeat.*

The *Easy Does It* Approach

Days 1–7	12-hour window	Low-carb ease-in breakfast, Low-carb ease-in lunch, Regular dinner
Days 8–14	10-hour window	Late low-carb ease-in breakfast or early low-carb ease-in lunch, Low-carb ease-in snack, Regular dinner
Days 15–21	8-hour window	Low-carb ease-in lunch, Regular dinner
Days 22–28	6-hour window	Low-carb ease-in lunch or low-carb ease-in snack, Regular dinner

In this approach, you're starting out in week 1 with three meals a day in a twelve-hour eating window. Notice that this plan includes some low-carb "ease-in" meals that will help your body lower insulin levels (*our bodies release less insulin in response to lower-carb meals*) while still eating three times a day at first. Have a low-carb breakfast, a low-carb lunch, and then eat the type of dinner that you're used to (dinner doesn't need to be low-carb unless you have already been living a low-carb lifestyle; remember that other than these low-carb ease-in meals, we aren't changing *what* we eat during the FAST Start, only *when* we eat).

Each week, you tighten up your eating window by a couple of hours, until you finally end up with a window of about six hours containing either two meals or a snack and a meal.

The *Steady Build* Approach

Days 1–7	8-hour window	Lunch, Dinner
Days 8–14	7-hour window	Lunch, Dinner
Days 15–21	6-hour window	Lunch or snack, Dinner
Days 22–28	5-hour window	Snack, Dinner

In this approach, you start off skipping breakfast on day 1, and BOOM! You're doing it! Stick to clean-fast-approved beverages all morning, and eat your typical lunch followed by your typical dinner within an eight-hour eating window.

Each week, you shorten your eating window by an hour,

and you end up in week 4 with an eating window of five hours that contains a snack and a meal.

The *Rip-Off-the-Band-Aid* Approach

Days 1–7	6-hour window	Lunch, Dinner
Days 8–14	6-hour window	Lunch or snack, Dinner
Days 15–21	5-hour window	Lunch or snack, Dinner
Days 22–28	4-hour window	Snack, Dinner

In this approach, you are maximizing your fasting time starting on day 1, with a six-hour window and therefore eighteen hours of daily fasting. The first week you skip breakfast and eat two meals, and over the course of weeks 2 and 3, you can choose to either eat lunch or transition lunch into more of a snack. In week 4, you end up with an eating window of four hours that contains a snack and a meal.

You may still have one nagging question after reading these plans:

Gin! What's the difference between a snack and a meal???

I've seen that question a lot. I want to encourage you to not get too hung up on terminology, but to decide if something qualifies as a meal, I ask myself this: If a friend invited me over for dinner and served this to me, would I consider it to have been an actual dinner? If not, it's probably a snack. Go with your gut here. However, since our goal every day is to eat until we are satisfied and not stuffed, it doesn't matter what you call it, now does it?

SETTING YOURSELF UP FOR SUCCESS: IDENTIFY YOUR *WHY*

Why did you pick up this book, and why did I create it? I don't just want to write a book that will sit on your shelf and collect dust. I also don't want you to start IF only to quit and get back on the diet train.

No, I want you to succeed. I want you to *be wildly successful. Beyond-your-greatest-dreams* levels of success. And to do that, you need a few things:

- » A positive mindset
- » Realistic expectations
- » Tools in your toolbox
- » The confidence that you have the power to make changes that make a difference long term
- » A powerful *why*

This chapter is for you to begin to craft your *why*.
I am sure you've heard this saying:

A journey of a thousand miles begins with one step.

Getting this book and committing to the FAST Start? That's an important first step on your journey. And you've taken that step.

But to get where you're going, you also have to know *where* you're going. If you want to go to the beach, you don't travel a thousand miles inland. No, you decide where you are going (the beach), and you point yourself in the *direction* of that destination.

That's what we are going to do now: figure out where you want to go.

If you're like most people, you're probably coming to IF with the goal of weight loss. That's certainly what brought me to IF: I was obese, and I was sick and tired of feeling sick and tired. I knew that along with weight loss, I would feel better in my body after I lost weight.

But what if I told you this . . . weight loss shouldn't be your primary destination.

Hang with me for a minute.

Is it *wrong* to have weight loss as your goal? Of course not. If you don't feel good in your body for whatever reason—and carrying around excess pounds *does not feel good*—then weight loss should absolutely be a big part of your *why*.

I want you to think *beyond* weight loss, though. Remember: I want you to succeed *beyond* your greatest dreams. I want you to be *wildly* successful. Maybe right now, all you can think about is looking down and seeing a smaller number on your scale display, or perhaps you dream of fitting into the smaller clothes you have stashed away for *one day*. Those are great dreams, and IF can make them happen for you.

But you deserve a lot more than simply having a body that has a lower gravitational pull.

Take a minute to check off all the items from the list that are a part of your *why*, and I've added blanks so you can add your own:

- ❏ I want to lose weight and keep it off
- ❏ I want to feel good in my body
- ❏ I want to fit into clothes that make me feel wonderful when I wear them
- ❏ I want to get off medications
- ❏ I want to lower my A1C
- ❏ I want to change my entire health trajectory so I age well and live a vibrant life
- ❏ I want to avoid diseases that are often linked to aging
- ❏ I want to be pain-free
- ❏ I want to have more physical endurance
- ❏ I want to maintain my muscle mass and become even stronger than I am now
- ❏ I want to enjoy foods again
- ❏ I want to cure my diet brain forever so I can stop trying to find yet another diet
- ❏ I want to be there for my family—my partner/spouse/ kids/grandkids—and for everyone I care about

- ❏ _____
  _____
- ❏ _____
  _____
- ❏ _____
  _____
- ❏ _____
  _____
- ❏ _____
  _____

You probably checked the first box: "I want to lose weight and keep it off." I don't blame you one bit! That is what brought me to IF as well.

The point of this exercise is that I want you to never forget all the *other* reasons you checked. Intermittent fasting changes lives in ways that have nothing to do with the number on the scale or the size of your clothes.

There are lots of ways to lose weight more quickly than IF. And I could tell you about all of them.

I'm going to say that again, for emphasis:

I could tell you about at least twenty ways to lose weight that would allow you to lose weight more quickly than you could with IF.

But we aren't here because we want the *quickest* weight loss we could find. Have you ever done a *lose-weight-quick!* program in the past that worked very well in the short term, but then you regained every pound you lost, plus more?

Me, too.

That's not what IF is. IF is slow and steady.

It's the *health plan* with a *side effect of weight loss.*

Don't allow a desire for quick weight loss to keep you from experiencing all the other potential benefits IF has to offer.

Look back over the list and reread what you checked. Summarize your reasons for wanting to live an intermittent fasting lifestyle into a few sentences or a paragraph, and write it down in the space provided here at the end of this chapter. Whenever you're struggling, you can come back and remember why you are an intermittent faster.

MY WHY:

I choose to live an intermittent fasting lifestyle because ____

_____

_____

_____

_____

_____

_____

_____

_____

_____

_____

_____

_____

_____

_____

_____

_____

DAY 0: PREPARING FOR SUCCESS BEFORE YOUR *IF* JOURNEY BEGINS

Welcome to day 0 . . . your IF journey starts tomorrow! Before you begin, you'll want to collect some baseline data. More about that in a minute.

But first—now that you have taken some time to identify your *why*, it's time to prepare yourself mentally for intermittent fasting success. Over the next four weeks, *intermittent fasting success* will be defined by one thing and one thing only:

Success is completing the 28-Day FAST Start.

As you get ready to begin, I want you to be very clear about the purpose of the FAST Start—what it *IS* and what it *ISN'T*:

» The purpose of the FAST Start *IS* to establish your daily intermittent fasting habit so your body adapts to fasting.
» The purpose of the FAST Start *IS NOT* weight loss.

I know that last one might be a surprise. *Wait a minute, Gin. I might not lose weight? What the what? Why on earth would I do this if I am not going to lose weight? Now you've lost me.*

Hang in there . . . let me explain.

On day 1 (or day 2, or day 10, or even day 17), your body is not yet skilled at tapping into your stored fat for fuel. You have to train your body to do that, and it takes more time than you might expect. I'll talk more about that in some of the daily lessons. For now, all you need to do is understand that your job is to release all expectations of weight loss . . . for now. There will be plenty of time to tweak for weight loss . . . AFTER the 28-Day FAST Start is over.

Before we go any further, I want you to make a commitment to yourself. Say this aloud (it might feel weird, but saying it out loud makes it more real):

I commit to completing the 28-Day FAST Start. This is a precious period of time that I am setting aside and protecting so my body can learn to do something new. I'm not going to stop in the middle of the FAST Start, but if I have a blip along the way, I'm not going to give up or think I need to start over. After the FAST Start is complete, I will have plenty of time to focus on any health or weight-loss goals I might have.

Hooray! You've just made a very important promise to yourself.

Now, let's talk about the nonnegotiable rules of the

FAST Start. I want you to also commit to each of these expectations. Check them off as you read them, and you may also want to read these aloud so they stick in your brain:

- ❑ Every day of the FAST Start, I will fast clean (plain water, unflavored sparkling water, black unflavored coffee, plain tea).
- ❑ During each daily fast, I will take time to reflect on the positive changes happening in my body.
- ❑ Within my daily eating window, I will eat until I am satisfied, and then I will stop.
- ❑ I will honor my "I've had enough" signals.
- ❑ I will stay off the scale until day 29.

Every day of your FAST Start, you'll reflect on the day, and part of that will include reminding yourself of those five daily expectations. As I said, they are nonnegotiable.

You may be wondering: Why is staying off the scale a nonnegotiable? This is where I want you to trust me and my years of experience.

I have seen a LOT of intermittent fasters get discouraged in the early days of their journey. Maybe they *know* I recommended that they not weigh, but they can't help themselves. One morning during their FAST Start, maybe they feel slim and strong and they *just know* that they have lost weight! So, they get on the scale, excited to see just how much they have lost . . .

. . . only to find their weight is UP from where it was when they started.

What happens then? Well, you can imagine what might go through your head if that happened to you:

This isn't working. I am gaining weight. Why am I doing this? Stupid IF. Not only is it hard, but I'm going in the wrong direction. Maybe I should buy that shake program again or try the weight-loss coaching plan my friend is selling.

Don't let that be you. *Stay OFF the scale during the FAST Start.* I promise you'll be glad you did.

If you think you can't do it, give your scale to a friend to keep for you until day 29. Make them promise not to give it back until day 29. That's how important it is to stay off the scale.

Once day 29 rolls around, I predict that you'll feel so much better that you won't want to stop IF, no matter what the scale says. Plus, by that point, you will understand that there are a great variety of tools in your IF toolbox so you can be confident that weight loss—if that's what you desire—is in your future.

Baseline data to collect on day 0:

DAY 0 . . . STARTING TOMORROW!

Date: _____

Starting weight: _____

Measurements: _____

    Bust or chest: _____

    Waist: _____

    Hips: _____

    Right thigh: _____

    Left thigh: _____

You can track other areas as well if you would like to. There are many places where you might want to measure yourself, or you might want to just take the five baseline measurements I list: the choice is yours. If you are not sure about *how* to measure yourself accurately, do a Google search or find an instructional video on YouTube that shows you proper measuring technique.

In addition to these measurements, take photos of yourself from the front, from the side, and from the back. If possible, get someone else to take them for you . . . but mirror selfies also work. Choose an outfit that is just a little too tight right now. You will wear the same exact clothes when you take new photos in twenty-eight days.

Keep one thing in mind: the data you record on day 0 is just that. It's simply information. Don't forget that the FAST Start period is for giving your body time to adjust to the clean fast, and you have committed to releasing *all* weight-loss expectations during this period.

Now that you have your baseline data recorded and you've made the commitment to yourself to begin (and complete) the FAST Start, it's time to get started! I am so excited for you to begin.

EXTRA CREDIT INFO

You may also want to have some blood work done, though this is optional. You don't need to wait to start IF until after you get this blood work done (because these markers change slowly over time), but if you're interested in this data, you should go ahead and set it up as soon as possible. Having baseline data from early in your IF journey related to some of your health markers can be powerful, because when you repeat the tests in a few months, you'll have confirmation of the powerful changes happening deep within your body.

If you're interested, I would recommend getting both an A1C and a fasting insulin test. You probably already know that an A1C is a great indicator of overall metabolic health, but perhaps you have never had a fasting insulin test, and it's likely your doctor has never even ordered one—they aren't standard practice. In *Fast. Feast. Repeat.*, I explain the concept of hyperinsulinemia (which roughly means "too much insulin") and why it's a problem, specifically as it relates to weight loss. Having high levels of insulin keeps your body from tapping into your fat stores effectively, which I will explain to you a bit more in the daily lesson about the clean fast on day 1.

There's also a great book called *Why We Get Sick* by Dr. Benjamin Bikman, which came out just over a year after I wrote *Fast. Feast. Repeat.* In it, he explains the common factor that links many major diseases—including cancer, diabetes, and Alzheimer's—and if you guessed the problem is unnaturally high levels of insulin, you would be right.

Here's what's exciting—fasting is the best way to get your insulin levels down. Therefore, knowing where you begin is great information to have.

What if your doctor won't order a fasting insulin test for you? Well, that would be a shame, and I would encourage you to recommend *Why We Get Sick* to your doctor, because this is information every doctor should have. But the good news is that in most states, you can take this into your own hands and order your own test through a third-party website. Google "order my own fasting insulin test" and see what you can find. Currently, I would be able to get this done for around twenty-five dollars by ordering the test online and then taking the paperwork to a participating lab near me.

WEEK 1 PLAN

Which of these did you choose for week 1 in the "Choose Your FAST Start Approach" chapter? (Look back to page 20 if you need to.)

☐ The *Easy Does It* Approach (twelve-hour window, low-carb ease-in breakfast and lunch, plus a regular dinner)

☐ The *Steady Build* Approach (eight-hour window, including lunch and dinner)

☐ The *Rip Off the Band-Aid* Approach (six-hour window, including lunch and dinner)

As your FAST Start progresses, never forget that these recommendations aren't carved in stone. You can reassess on any day and ease up or tighten up your window as needed or desired.

You are in charge at all times: These three approaches are all general guidelines that you can choose to follow or adapt as needed. You know yourself better than anyone else does, and I want you to always feel empowered to chart your own course.

DAY 1: NAIL THE CLEAN FAST: *WHY* AND *HOW*

Today's Date: _____

PLANNING FOR A SUCCESSFUL DAY 1

Today, I am following

- ❏ The *Easy Does It* Approach (twelve-hour window, low-carb ease-in breakfast and lunch, plus a regular dinner)
- ❏ The *Steady Build* Approach (eight-hour window, including lunch and dinner)
- ❏ The *Rip Off the Band-Aid* Approach (six-hour window, including lunch and dinner)

My personal goal(s) for today: _____

_____

_____

_____

_____

Daily Lesson from Gin: Nail the clean fast: *why* and *how*.

This is not one of those short-and-sweet daily lessons, because it is too important. To fully understand and embrace the recommendations for the clean fast, you need to be clear on *why* you are fasting. On day 3, I'll explain the difference between fasting and low-calorie dieting, and it's important.

For today, though, know this:

You're either fasting clean, or you aren't fasting.

And to put it another way:

You're either fasting clean, or you're doing a low-calorie diet.

And a low-calorie diet isn't fasting.

This is such a foundational topic that I have two complete chapters in *Fast. Feast. Repeat.* that explain why we fast clean and how to make sure we are fasting clean, and these chapters are twenty-eight pages in total. So, you can see that the part I am sharing here is not a substitute for reading those chapters.

Those chapters also include a discussion of the scientific rationale behind the three clean fasting goals, along with links to resources and references (all listed in the references section of *Fast. Feast. Repeat.*).

So, today I am going to give you the basics only and trust that you will take the time to read the clean fast chapters of *Fast. Feast. Repeat.* later. Don't skip it—I firmly believe that when you fully understand the science behind these recommendations, you'll be more likely to embrace the guidelines.

By having the full understanding of the clean fast, you also won't be fooled by marketing claims such as *"Buy my fasting beverage! It's sweet and delicious and perfectly safe for the fast!"* or *"I have some fasting tea I want to sell you! It is fruity and delicious, and it will get you through the fast!"* or *"Buy these fasting bars! It's just like fasting except you're eating!"* or *"Buy my fasting supplement! It has all sorts of additives and it's perfect for fasting, and you also need it!"*

Side note: You don't need to buy any special fasting beverages. There are no special fasting coffees or teas you need. There are no fasting bars that will help you fast (*eating is not fasting*). There are no fasting supplements you need.

No, no, no, and *no*.

So, let's get started so you understand the basics.

During the clean fast, these are our main goals:

1. Keep insulin levels as low as possible during the fast;
2. Tap into our own fat stores for fuel; and
3. Experience increased autophagy and all the upcycling that comes along with it. *(You may not yet know what autophagy is or why you should care . . . but I am going to explain it to you on day 5, so stay tuned!)*

Once we understand the GOALS of the clean fast, we can understand how to make those things happen:

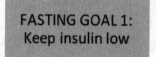

FASTING GOAL 1:
Keep insulin low

BY: Avoiding anything that tastes sweet or food-like

Why do we care about insulin? You may have only ever heard of insulin in the context of diabetes, and maybe you have a vague understanding of insulin as something that diabetics need to lower their blood sugar. But there's a lot more to it than that.

If your pancreas is functioning properly, your body releases insulin anytime you eat (or anytime your body *thinks* you are eating . . . more about that in a moment). Insulin is required to keep your blood sugar from rising too quickly, that's true. Insulin is, in fact, a storage hormone, and it helps our cells take in the glucose from our blood and store it away for later.

Insulin is also *antilipolytic*, meaning it works against fat burning. It's important to understand what I am saying here: **If you have high levels of insulin, that is actively working against fat burning. If you're in storage mode (which goes along with high insulin levels), you aren't in fat-burning mode (which requires low insulin levels).**

While fasting, you want to avoid anything that makes your body release additional insulin beyond what it needs to keep your blood glucose within its normal range.

Our bodies have a nifty mechanism called the *cephalic phase insulin response*, or CPIR. When your taste buds sense food flavors, this message goes to your brain. Your brain understands this message: *Food is coming in! We need more INSULIN!* Even before the glucose can hit your bloodstream, the CPIR causes your pancreas to release insulin to prepare for what's coming.

Here's the problem in today's society, however. Thanks to modern chemistry, not all food flavors are telling our brains the true story. A diet soda is one example of this. Flavored coffee beans, lemon in our water, flavored herbal teas . . . those are a few other examples. Each of those may have zero calories, but the brain has no idea about that. All the brain knows is this:

Food flavor incoming! Need more insulin NOW!

While fasting clean, we want to avoid the CPIR at all costs. Flavors matter.

To learn more about this topic, you'll find examples of

the research in the clean fast chapters of *Fast. Feast. Repeat.* It's fascinating to understand, and it changes the way you look at a diet soda forever.

1

You may wonder: If we are going to avoid "flavors," why can we have black coffee and plain tea? Don't they have a "flavor"? They do, but they have a bitter flavor profile, which doesn't stimulate an insulin response.

SUMMARY: To keep insulin low, we avoid anything that makes our bodies think food is coming in.

WE SAY YES TO:
- Plain water, with no flavors or enhancers added (including fruits or fruit essences of any type)
- Plain sparkling or mineral water, with no flavors or enhancers added
- Black coffee, with no added flavors or milky additives (this includes avoiding *all* animal- or plant-based milks, creams, or creamers)
- Plain tea, such as black tea or green tea, with no added flavors or milky additives (this includes avoiding *all* animal- or plant-based milks, creams, or creamers)

WE SAY NO TO:
- Food
- Flavored water or flavored sparkling water
- Herbal teas that are fruity, flavored, or sweet in any way
- Matcha tea
- Flavored coffee
- Sweeteners of all types
- All food flavors (this includes things like herbs, spices, vinegars, etc.)

- Natural or artificial flavors
- Bottled or packaged coffee or tea products that contain ANY ingredients other than coffee or tea and water (particularly watch out for the sneaky flavor-adding citric acid)

FASTING GOAL 2: Tap into our own fat stores for fuel		BY: Avoiding anything that provides an external fuel source, such as fat in coffee or exogenous ketone supplements

This one is a lot less complicated than fasting goal 1. All you need to do is ask yourself this question: *Do you want to burn the fat from your body, or do you want to burn fuel you're taking in?* During the clean fast, we want to burn the fat from our bodies, or the fuel that is already inside of us, and to do that, we must avoid taking in new sources of fuel.

SUMMARY: To tap into our own fat stores for fuel, we avoid anything that is a source of fuel for our bodies.

WE SAY YES TO:
- Plain water, with no flavors or enhancers added (including fruits of any type)
- Plain sparkling or mineral water, with no flavors or enhancers added
- Black coffee, with no added flavors or milky additives (this includes avoiding *all* animal- or plant-based milks, creams, or creamers)
- Plain tea, such as black tea or green tea, with no added flavors or milky additives (this includes avoiding *all* animal- or plant-based milks, creams, or creamers)

WE SAY NO TO:

- Food
- Butter, MCT oil, or coconut oil in our beverages or any oil as a supplement
- All creams or creamers, whether animal- or plant-based
- Exogenous ketone supplements

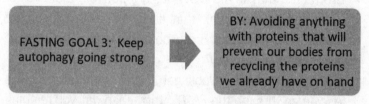

FASTING GOAL 3: Keep autophagy going strong

BY: Avoiding anything with proteins that will prevent our bodies from recycling the proteins we already have on hand

I'll explain autophagy in more detail on day 5. Once you understand what autophagy is, you'll understand why we don't want to stop it from happening. Autophagy is upregulated when we are fasting, and our bodies are able to do important cellular housekeeping and recycling. What stops autophagy? Eating, but also consuming sources of protein. If protein is coming in, we don't need to recycle old junky proteins.

SUMMARY: To keep autophagy going strong, we avoid anything that contains protein.

WE SAY YES TO:

- Plain water, with no flavors or enhancers added (including fruits of any type)
- Plain sparkling or mineral water, with no flavors or enhancers added
- Black coffee, with no added flavors or milky additives (this includes avoiding *all* animal- or plant-based milks, creams, or creamers)

- Plain tea, such as black tea or green tea, with no added flavors or milky additives (this includes avoiding *all* animal- or plant-based milks, creams, or creamers)

WE SAY NO TO:
- Food
- Broth (You may think, *DUH, it's a food.* Yes, that is true, but some people think that it doesn't count for some reason. Well, it does. Broth not only tastes like food, it also contains protein.)
- Supplements such as collagen, pre-workouts, or BCAAs

As you go through the FAST Start, each day you're going to commit to fasting clean. You can always go back to page 18 to check the graphic that illustrates the clean fast.

EXTRA CREDIT READING
Chapters 4 and 5 of *Fast. Feast. Repeat.* Those two chapters explain why and how we fast clean in a lot more detail, with links to all the research that the clean fast is founded on.

DAILY INSPIRATION SPOTLIGHT:
Shana Hussin, Kauauna, Wisconsin
Intermittent Fasting Stories guest, episode 109

How long has she been an intermittent faster? Between three and four years.
I am a registered dietitian, in the field for twenty-three years. For much of that time, I taught conventional guidelines of "eat less and move more" and "eat frequently to keep your energy up" and "make sure to include many healthy whole grains, fruits, and veggies at all your meals." My students,

1

patients, and clients struggled after I gave them these recommendations, and for good reason. They were horrible guidelines that made most people sick and fat. In 2016, my son became very ill with ulcerative colitis (inflammatory bowel disease), and we were thrown into the conventional medical system, with conventional treatments for the first time in our lives. I was not impressed. I was made to feel I should not question anything at any time, let alone harsh treatments that would suppress my son's immune system long term. We went through years of illness and heartache. I knew there had to be a better way, and I eventually found a treatment that healed him on my own. Throughout this time, I did a deep dive into natural nutrition treatments and what caused chronic disease. I read The Obesity Code and Delay, Don't Deny in 2018, and EVERYTHING shifted. I had left the conventional nutrition system because I no longer believed in what I was teaching, and I finally figured out why my patients had struggled with their weight and health for SO LONG. The education for dietitians was severely flawed. I implemented IF in my own life as an experiment because I didn't believe it was actually healthy. Boy, was I WRONG! I immediately had less bloating, more energy, more time, less stress, and just felt BETTER. For the first time in ten years, my chronic canker sores started to heal. I had never had a big weight issue, but weight management became virtually effortless, and I stopped constantly thinking about food and snacking. I opened my online nutrition therapy practice within the year, wrote my book called Fast to Heal, and even started my own podcast, which now consistently ranks in the top hundred of all nutrition podcasts. I currently teach online courses to reverse insulin resistance, where intermittent fasting is a huge strategy to adapt, along with proper meal order and therapeutic carb restriction. I help people reverse their insulin resistance, obesity, fatty liver, prediabetes and type 2 diabetes, and blood pressure and lipid issues every single day! Rather than adding in more medications, they are getting OFF of them! I am so blessed to be able to share these simple approaches that change lives and help people heal for good. My professional and personal lives have completely changed due to IF, and I live the dream of helping others do the same. I typically eat twice a day and fast sixteen to eighteen hours most days. I fast twenty-four hours one or two times a month. I maintain my weight and am not looking to lose any. I am at an ideal body composition with no medical issues, and my strategies are for maintenance. I am one of the 12 percent of Americans who are metabolically healthy. I focus on balanced meals and a low-carb approach. I sleep well and have a more regular menstrual cycle at forty-seven than I did at seventeen. I do not snack or have anything sugary in between meals or in the evening.

ADVICE FROM SHANA
Intermittent fasting is the single most potent strategy to keep insulin levels low throughout much of the day, which helps us burn fat, become metabolically flexible, and avoid chronic lifestyle disease!

YOU HAVE ALL THE TOOLS YOU NEED TO SUCCEED. ENJOY YOUR DAY! YOU'VE GOT THIS.

HOW DID IT GO?
IT'S TIME TO REFLECT ON DAY 1.

TODAY (CHECK ALL THAT APPLY):

- ❏ I fasted clean (plain water, unflavored sparkling water, black unflavored coffee, plain tea)
- ❏ During the fast, I took time to reflect on the positive changes happening in my body
- ❏ Within my eating window, I ate until I was satisfied, and then I stopped
- ❏ I honored my "I've had enough" signals
- ❏ I stayed off the scale

FAST CHECK-IN

Rate the difficulty of today's fast on a scale from 1 to 10 (circle one):

1　2　3　4　5　6　7　8　9　**10**

(Today was easy! I sailed right through it.)　　　(Today was HARD! I struggled.)

During today's fast, I felt _____

_____

_____

_____

_____

_____

(*examples: exhilarated, hopeful, hungry, uncomfortable, bored, etc.*)

I used these strategies to manage my feelings today (check all that apply and add your own):

❏ I remembered my *why*
❏ I stayed busy
❏ I enjoyed a clean-fast-safe beverage
❏ I went on a walk
❏ I imagined my body tapping into my fat stores for fuel
❏ _____
  _____
❏ _____
  _____
❏ _____
  _____

EATING WINDOW CHECK-IN

Eating Window Length Goal: _____ hours
Actual Eating Window Length: _____ hours

How do I feel about today's eating window?

_____
_____
_____
_____
_____
_____
_____
_____
_____

What went well? Was there anything that I struggled with during my eating window? _____

_____

_____

_____

_____

_____

_____

_____

_____

_____

_____

TODAY'S NSVS, OR NON-SCALE VICTORIES

One of the most powerful things we can do is acknowledge our Non-Scale Victories (NSVs). These can be physical (*pain reduction, better energy, mental clarity, etc.*) or emotional (*freedom around food, confidence, etc.*).

What were today's NSVs? _____

_____

_____

_____

_____

_____

_____

_____

_____

REFLECTIONS

Today, I listened to my body when I: _____

_____

_____

_____

_____

_____

_____

_____

_____

Today's *AHA!* moment(s): _____

_____

_____

_____

Something that is on my mind: _____

_____

_____

_____

PREPARING FOR SUCCESS

Goal(s) and/or strategies for tomorrow: _____

_____

_____

_____

_____

DAY 2: BUT I REALLY CAN'T DRINK MY COFFEE BLACK, GIN. *I. CAN. NOT.*

Today's Date: _____

PLANNING FOR A SUCCESSFUL DAY 2

2

Today, I am following

❏ The *Easy Does It* Approach (twelve-hour window, low-carb ease-in breakfast and lunch, plus a regular dinner)
❏ The *Steady Build* Approach (eight-hour window, including lunch and dinner)
❏ The *Rip Off the Band-Aid* Approach (six-hour window, including lunch and dinner)

My personal goal(s) for today: _____

_____

_____

_____

_____

_____

Daily Lesson from Gin: But I REALLY can't drink my coffee black, Gin. *I. Can. Not.*

Today, we are going to tackle one of the most contentious topics in the clean fasting world: black coffee versus what I like to call "hot milkshakes."

And maybe you don't drink coffee, but you love tea with

a little something added to it. Or you love flavored sparkling water. Or gum. Or mints. And you don't want to give them up.

The lessons here relating to coffee can apply to your tea, or your sparkling water, or whatever it is you're used to having that you think you need and you don't want to give up.

So, I'm going to talk about coffee today, since that is the number one stumbling block I hear about from new IFers, but apply these lessons to your own situation. You can replace the word *coffee* with whatever you're struggling with.

Switching to black coffee was a big freaking deal for me.

I can't express how much I enjoyed my daily lattes. I loved them so much that I bought a fancy coffee machine for my classroom that allowed me to produce lattes in minutes by popping in a couple of cartridges and pushing a button. I would add my zero-calorie sweetener of choice and enjoy my delicious hot milkshake. It was such an important ritual that whenever I would walk toward that corner of my classroom, my students knew I was making another latte.

When I started fasting consistently in 2014, I instinctively knew that milk wasn't part of any fast (since it is the perfect food for baby mammals who are growing quickly), so I stopped with the lattes (most of the time . . .). But because I was so thoroughly steeped in the calories in / calories out mindset, I didn't see the harm in adding Vanilla Crème Stevia and a dash of cinnamon to my multiple daily cups of coffee. My coffee was still sweet and delicious, and it still had that "hot milkshake" quality I was looking for, but with zero calories. What could go wrong?

Then I read *The Obesity Code* in the spring of 2016. In

it, Dr. Jason Fung explained the cephalic phase insulin response, also known as CPIR. As you remember from what I explained to you in the lesson about the clean fast on day 1, we want to avoid anything that causes our bodies to release more insulin during the fast, since our goal is to keep insulin low so our bodies can access our fat stores.

I remember the emotions I felt when I learned about the CPIR.

What the what??? You've got to be kidding me! Well, *I* CANNOT drink black coffee. Nope. I guess coffee is OUT.

If I couldn't drink my coffee hot-milkshake style, I wasn't going to have coffee at all. So there.

I lasted for a couple of days on the "no coffee" wagon, but I really missed coffee (and it wasn't just the caffeine withdrawals speaking). I missed the ritual of coffee, and coffee's soothing aroma.

I decided right then and there that I would put on my big-girl pants and drink my coffee black.

The first day, I am not going to lie, it was awful. I held my nose and drank it. I did the same thing the next day and the next and the next.

And I didn't die.

A funny thing happened in a week or so: I didn't hate it anymore. I was a black coffee drinker! My taste buds had adjusted. What kind of (*black coffee*) magic was this?

An even funnier thing happened a few months later. My eating window was open, and I decided I would have my favorite hot milkshake to celebrate. The holidays were approaching, and my favorite seasonal flavor was available. I placed my order and excitedly took the first sip.

What.

I didn't like it. Not even a little bit.

2

You see, once my taste buds adjusted to black coffee, it turns out I *prefer* it that way.

Huh. Who'd've thunk it?

You may be reading this and thinking that this is all well and good, but *you* can't do it. Plus, you saw a YouTube video that said it's fine to add ___ to your coffee (or to your tea, or to your water), so you're going to conveniently forget that I mentioned black coffee. How could a little _____ (fill in the blank with whatever) really make a difference?

Trust me, new IFer. It does.

When you read the clean fast chapters in *Fast. Feast. Repeat.*, you will read about something I call the Clean Fast Challenge. During the FAST Start, one of our nonnegotiables for success is committing to the clean fast. So, if you're here doing the FAST Start, I expect you to take the Clean Fast Challenge.

You know how your best elementary school teachers had eyes in the back of their heads and they knew what was going on? Or how Santa was always watching throughout the year, but especially in December? Ahem. Pretend that I am watching you, new IFer.

And I am watching you as you NAIL the clean fast, every single day of your FAST Start.

Even if you don't yet believe that the clean fast matters, can you trust me enough to listen to my years of experience here? If you don't, trust the forty-three IFers in the clean fast chapter of *Fast. Feast. Repeat.* who explained how the clean fast made a difference to them. Or the thousands of clean fasters from around the world, hundreds of whom have told their stories on the *Intermittent Fasting Stories* podcast. One day, you'll be a believer, but for now, believe those of us who have walked the path before you.

To succeed with the clean fast, you have two choices:

- You can skip coffee (or tea) entirely if you want. It's perfectly fine to fast with plain water only. *If you're worried about caffeine withdrawal, a caffeine pill might be an option to help you get over the hump.*
- Or, you can hold your nose and drink it black until that magical day your taste buds adjust, just as mine did.

I KNOW you can do it.

Thousands of other successful IFers have done it, and you can, too.

EXTRA CREDIT READING

The end of chapter 5 of *Fast. Feast. Repeat.* Find the pages that explain the Clean Fast Challenge and also the ones that contain stories from dozens of IFers who discovered the amazing difference the clean fast made for them.

================================

DAILY INSPIRATION SPOTLIGHT:

Renee Jocson, Normal, Illinois
Intermittent Fasting Stories guest, episode 267

How long has she been an intermittent faster? *Between two and three years.*

My first experience with IF was in 2011 when my husband and I were preparing to make our first trip to Hawaii. We were also doing P90X, and we got RIPPED! I'm talking amazing abs! Unfortunately, I can take things to the extreme, and

I wasn't very educated in IF. I would fast, but never really feasted. I fasted and restricted. And, oh boy, did that do a number on my body and on my gut! (Note to reader: DON'T DO THIS.) Quickly on the heels of this calorie/nutrient deficit in my body, my parents' health declined drastically, requiring my help, my job as a pediatric mental health nurse blew up exponentially, I enrolled in an online program to become a health coach, and menopause hit hard. I gained weight, was terminally bloated (you know the look. . . . where your arms don't go down nicely on your sides . . . you look a bit like a hulk), I had an "upper belly" that I couldn't suck in, and I was miserable. I did go to a functional medicine doctor for a lot of my issues, which helped me lose a little weight, but I couldn't regain the body I loved. I've always been small, so carrying even fifteen extra pounds shows up big on my small frame. In late 2019 / early 2020, I decided to give IF a try again. I had an eight-hour window. I read/heard that you can have butter and MCT oil in your coffee and still be in the fasting state. Whew! Did I ever love that coffee. But I wasn't losing weight (incidentally, I didn't know much about autophagy, either). I believed in IF and recommended it to the women in my coaching practice, but I wasn't seeing results in my own body. My best friend, Stacy, read Gin's book Delay, Don't Deny, *implemented IF, and started losing weight for the first time in her life. She told me about the clean fast. I was totally motivated by her success, so I cut out the "yummiest coffee in the whole world" and shortened my window. I know I can have the yummy coffee in my window, but it's not the same as first thing in the morning. Within six months, I was at my ideal weight. Today, I wear a size smaller than I did in 2020, I have more energy than I know what to do with, and I revamped my coaching practice*

(Your Food Fight LLC) from focusing on autoimmune disorders to helping middle-aged women lose weight and keep it off! The best part is seeing other women realize their weight-loss goals. My philosophy has become—if we can take extra weight out of the picture (through IF), then we can start to uncover all the other things that lead to the weight gain in the first place. As a small woman, the best part for me is that through autophagy, I am preventing chronic illness, plus my body fits my small frame, and my arms lie down at my sides!

2

ADVICE FROM RENEE

Two thoughts: No matter the size of your window, you must nourish your body. Make sure you're getting nutrient-dense foods—vegetables, fruit, protein, and healthy fats. Fasting + restricting doesn't work. If you fast, you must feast.

**YOU HAVE ALL THE TOOLS YOU NEED TO SUCCEED.
ENJOY YOUR DAY! YOU'VE GOT THIS.**

HOW DID IT GO?
IT'S TIME TO REFLECT ON DAY 2.

TODAY (CHECK ALL THAT APPLY):

- ❏ I fasted clean (plain water, unflavored sparkling water, black unflavored coffee, plain tea)
- ❏ During the fast, I took time to reflect on the positive changes happening in my body
- ❏ Within my eating window, I ate until I was satisfied, and then I stopped
- ❏ I honored my "I've had enough" signals
- ❏ I stayed off the scale

FAST CHECK-IN

Rate the difficulty of today's fast on a scale from 1 to 10 (circle one):

1 2 3 4 5 6 7 8 9 **10**

(Today was easy! I sailed right through it.)   (Today was HARD! I struggled.)

During today's fast, I felt _____

_____

_____

_____

_____

_____

(*examples: exhilarated, hopeful, hungry, uncomfortable, bored, etc.*)

I used these strategies to manage my feelings today (check all that apply and add your own):

- ❑ I remembered my *why*
- ❑ I stayed busy
- ❑ I enjoyed a clean-fast-safe beverage
- ❑ I went on a walk
- ❑ I imagined my body tapping into my fat stores for fuel
- ❑ _____
  _____
- ❑ _____
  _____
- ❑ _____
  _____

EATING WINDOW CHECK-IN

Eating Window Length Goal: _____ hours
Actual Eating Window Length: _____ hours

How do I feel about today's eating window?

_____
_____
_____
_____
_____
_____
_____
_____
_____
_____

What went well? Was there anything that I struggled with during my eating window? _____

_____

_____

_____

_____

_____

_____

_____

_____

_____

TODAY'S NSVS, OR NON-SCALE VICTORIES

One of the most powerful things we can do is acknowledge our Non-Scale Victories (NSVs). These can be physical (*pain reduction, better energy, mental clarity, etc.*) or emotional (*freedom around food, confidence, etc.*).

What were today's NSVs? _____

_____

_____

_____

_____

_____

_____

_____

_____

REFLECTIONS

Today, I listened to my body when I: _____

_____

_____

_____

_____

_____

_____

_____

Today's *AHA!* moment(s): _____

_____

_____

_____

Something that is on my mind: _____

_____

_____

_____

PREPARING FOR SUCCESS

Goal(s) and/or strategies for tomorrow: _____

_____

_____

_____

_____

DAY 3: HOW IS FASTING DIFFERENT FROM A LOW-CALORIE DIET?

Today's Date: _____

PLANNING FOR A SUCCESSFUL DAY 3

Today, I am following

- ❏ The *Easy Does It* Approach (twelve-hour window, low-carb ease-in breakfast and lunch, plus a regular dinner)
- ❏ The *Steady Build* Approach (eight-hour window, including lunch and dinner)
- ❏ The *Rip Off the Band-Aid* Approach (six-hour window, including lunch and dinner)

My personal goal(s) for today: _____

_____

_____

_____

_____

Daily Lesson from Gin: How is fasting different from a low-calorie diet?

When I first began living an intermittent fasting lifestyle in 2014, everything I read about fasting explained that the reason fasting "worked" was because it made it easier for us to eat fewer calories, and since we were eating fewer calories, we would lose weight. Calories in / calories out.

Then, in 2016, I read *The Obesity Code* by Dr. Jason Fung, and I realized . . . BOY, were we all wrong about the calorie thing. It turns out, our bodies are a lot more complicated than the idea of calories in / calories out would lead us to believe.

We have all heard that theory: eat less, move more, and you will lose weight. In fact, I bet you've lost weight using that approach before. I know I have. I counted calories and lost weight.

It's all just a math equation, right? Well, no. Not even close.

You see, when we restrict what we are eating through a typical low-calorie diet where we are eating frequent small meals throughout the day, we do lose weight . . . at first. Then, weight loss begins to slow and often even stops. You start to feel miserable, you're STARVING, and then you find yourself eating everything in your pantry or fridge.

Just like that, the diet is over, and you are mad at yourself for what feels like a lack of willpower. The good news is that it never was about your willpower—it was that you were working against your body without even realizing it.

To understand, think about what I taught you on day 1:

If your pancreas is functioning properly, your body releases insulin anytime you eat (or anytime your body thinks you are eating). Insulin is required to keep your blood sugar from rising too quickly. Insulin is, in fact, a storage hormone, and it helps our cells take in the glucose from our blood and store it away for later.

*Insulin is also antilipolytic, meaning it works against fat burning. It's important to understand what I am saying here: **If you have high levels of insulin, that is actively working against fat burning. If you're*** *in storage mode (which goes along with high insulin levels), you aren't in fat-burning mode (which requires low insulin levels).*

When you were following one of those low-calorie diets with frequent small meals, every time you had one of those meals or snacks (or when you drank a zero-calorie beverage), your body released insulin in response. The constant release of insulin kept you in storage mode rather than letting your body get into fat-burning mode. When your blood sugar would drop (after the insulin came in) you got HUNGRY, and you would respond by having another small snack or low-calorie beverage. This kept you trapped on the blood sugar roller coaster all day long, and the constant flow of insulin kept you from tapping into your fat stores to fuel your body once the fuel from your tiny meals and snacks ran out. Hello, HANGRY.

Still, though, you powered through as long as you could. You were seeing weight loss, and you knew that you just needed to keep going. You kept white-knuckling through each day.

Behind the scenes, however, your body knew it wasn't well fueled, and the high levels of insulin from all those meals, snacks, and beverages kept you from burning much fat. Your body may have even turned to valuable muscle mass out of desperation. And then your body began to get even more concerned.

Our bodies have one goal: to keep us alive.

Your body didn't know that you were trying to lose weight and that you were restricting your foods on purpose. Instead, your body thought something terrible was happening, and the only thing it could do to save your life was to slow your metabolic rate, while at the same time sending you powerful "EAT SOME FOOD WHEN YOU CAN!" messages.

And just like that, the conventional low-calorie diet advice failed you once again.

You were able to white-knuckle your way through the *calories in* side of the equation for only so long before your body slowed your metabolic rate, which changed the *calories out* side of the equation. And to top it off, your body sent powerful signals to increase how much you were eating. *Calories in* went up at the same time that *calories out* went down.

You know how it ended. You regained more weight than you lost, and your metabolism was in worse shape than when you started. You were probably also flabbier, thanks to the loss in muscle mass.

The good news is that fasting changes this equation in powerful ways.

When you are fasting clean, your body doesn't need to release so much insulin all day long (though we always have a baseline level of insulin), and when insulin levels are lower, your body is able to tap into your fat stores for fuel.

When you're tapping into your fat stores for fuel during your daily fast, your body is happily well fueled. Because you're well fueled, your body doesn't need to slow your metabolic rate. Your body doesn't need to burn valuable muscle tissue, meaning you lose fat rather than muscle.

All of this doesn't happen on day 1 of your FAST Start, however. It takes time for your body to become what we call *fat adapted*. I will fully explain the concept of being fat adapted on day 9. Until you are fat adapted, keep in mind that you will *not* be well fueled during your fast, and you may experience both brain fog and tiredness, as well as increased hunger signals. This is all normal, and I promise it will get better after your body realizes how to access all the stored fuel that is already on your body, waiting to be tapped.

EXTRA CREDIT READING

You probably want to take a deeper dive on this topic, and I highly recommend that you do. Read the Introduction of *Fast. Feast. Repeat.* In it, you'll find a discussion of the ways low-calorie dieting has failed us, with links to the science that explains it. You'll learn about the Minnesota Starvation Experiment and the Biggest Loser Study, and then you'll finally understand the flaws in calories in / calories out. You'll realize that you didn't fail diets . . . diets failed YOU.

DAILY INSPIRATION SPOTLIGHT:
Tiffany Sayles, Gadsden, Alabama
Intermittent Fasting Stories guest, episode 137

How long has she been an intermittent faster? *Between three and four years.*

My journey with IF began December 2017 (during what I think of as my "ledge moment"). It was a few weeks before my fortieth birthday, and it was a pivotal point in my life. I knew that I could not continue to navigate life as I had been. I also realized that I had lived for everyone except for myself. It was time for me to prioritize myself. Holistic health was my goal. Although I had always been overweight, I strived to live a healthy lifestyle. I played basketball in middle school and also was in the marching band for six years. Despite my weight, my body was faithful to me. However, as I neared forty, I knew that I could not continue to take it for granted. At 324 pounds, I needed to make some additional changes. I was already actively working out five days a week but needed to modify my eating patterns. I began a 16:8 protocol and eventually worked up to a 20:4. When I was successfully committed to the IF protocols, the weight would consistently drop. I also completed some ADF weeks and 23:1. [Note from Gin: To learn more about ADF, read the ADF chapter in Fast. Feast. Repeat.*] 20:4 always worked best for me. The IF lifestyle has enhanced my life holistically. Although I continue to have more pounds to lose, my labs are always great, and I feel better than I did before forty, and I continue to SHINE. Health is greater than a number on the scale or seeking the latest diet fad. It is about honoring your whole self to include the physical, emotional, and spiritual. As I continue to adhere to the IF lifestyle, my health continues to improve, and I have influenced others to begin the journey. Consistency is key, and I recognize that this is truly not a sprint but a marathon. I am proud to say five years later, I am still running the IF race. It is a daily choice to get up and continue the work of a healthy lifestyle. I am worth it!*

3

ADVICE FROM TIFFANY

Consider and remember the why *of choosing this lifestyle. The scale will change, but it can't be your focus. We fast every day, and it is up to you to decide what fasting protocol will work for you to achieve the results you would like to see. Everyone's body and journey is different. Study yourself and what works for you. Gin has also provided so many resources to help each of us walk out this journey. IF is not a diet but a commitment and consistent decision to choose better health. No matter if you are new to this lifestyle or returning to it, you can start right now. Remember, it is not how or when you start but how you finish. We can do this—together!*

YOU HAVE ALL THE TOOLS YOU NEED TO SUCCEED. ENJOY YOUR DAY! YOU'VE GOT THIS.

HOW DID IT GO?
IT'S TIME TO REFLECT ON DAY 3.

TODAY (CHECK ALL THAT APPLY):

❏ I fasted clean (plain water, unflavored sparkling water, black unflavored coffee, plain tea)

❏ During the fast, I took time to reflect on the positive changes happening in my body

❏ Within my eating window, I ate until I was satisfied, and then I stopped

❏ I honored my "I've had enough" signals

❏ I stayed off the scale

FAST CHECK-IN

Rate the difficulty of today's fast on a scale from 1 to 10 (circle one):

1 2 3 4 5 6 7 8 9 **10**

(Today was easy! I sailed right through it.)   (Today was HARD! I struggled.)

During today's fast, I felt _____

_____

_____

_____

_____

_____

(*examples: exhilarated, hopeful, hungry, uncomfortable, bored, etc.*)

I used these strategies to manage my feelings today (check all that apply and add your own):

- ❏ I remembered my *why*
- ❏ I stayed busy
- ❏ I enjoyed a clean-fast-safe beverage
- ❏ I went on a walk
- ❏ I imagined my body tapping into my fat stores for fuel
- ❏ _____
  _____
- ❏ _____
  _____
- ❏ _____
  _____

EATING WINDOW CHECK-IN

Eating Window Length Goal: _____ hours
Actual Eating Window Length: _____ hours

How do I feel about today's eating window?

_____
_____
_____
_____
_____
_____
_____
_____
_____
_____

What went well? Was there anything that I struggled with during my eating window? _____

_____

_____

_____

_____

_____

_____

_____

_____

_____

_____

TODAY'S NSVS, OR NON-SCALE VICTORIES

One of the most powerful things we can do is acknowledge our Non-Scale Victories (NSVs). These can be physical (*pain reduction, better energy, mental clarity, etc.*) or emotional (*freedom around food, confidence, etc.*).

What were today's NSVs? _____

_____

_____

_____

_____

_____

_____

_____

_____

REFLECTIONS

Today, I listened to my body when I: _____

_____

_____

_____

_____

_____

_____

_____

_____

Today's *AHA!* moment(s): _____

_____

_____

_____

Something that is on my mind: _____

_____

_____

_____

_____

PREPARING FOR SUCCESS

Goal(s) and/or strategies for tomorrow: _____

_____

_____

_____

_____

DAY 4: HEALTH BENEFITS— WHAT DOES THE SCIENCE SAY?

Today's Date: _____

PLANNING FOR A SUCCESSFUL DAY 4

Today, I am following

- ❏ The *Easy Does It* Approach (twelve-hour window, low-carb ease-in breakfast and lunch, plus a regular dinner)
- ❏ The *Steady Build* Approach (eight-hour window, including lunch and dinner)
- ❏ The *Rip Off the Band-Aid* Approach (six-hour window, including lunch and dinner)

4

My personal goal(s) for today: _____

_____

_____

_____

_____

Daily Lesson from Gin: Health benefits—what does the science say?

Most of us come to intermittent fasting because we are looking for weight loss; however, when we think of intermittent fasting solely as a weight-loss approach, it's like looking at the tip of an iceberg and not understanding that the true bulk of that iceberg lies beneath the surface where you can't see it. If intermittent fasting is the iceberg, the weight loss is the part you can see above the surface, but everything else that IF can do for you is below. Just because you can't see it, that doesn't mean it isn't huge and powerful.

I like to call intermittent fasting the health plan with a side effect of weight loss. Here are some of the things that IF has the potential to do for you, and as you read over this list, you'll see that living an intermittent fasting lifestyle is about *so much more than weight loss*.

- **Fasting combats hyperinsulinemia**—What is *hyperinsulinemia*, and why do we care? High levels of insulin—also known as *hyperinsulinemia*—is connected to many negative health outcomes and is also linked to obesity. The best way to bring down insulin levels? The clean fast.
- **Fasting can prevent and reverse metabolic syndrome**—Metabolic syndrome is defined by a cluster of symptoms, including obesity (particularly abdominal obesity), insulin resistance, elevated cholesterol, and high blood pressure. Fasting has been shown to be beneficial for each one of those defining characteristics of metabolic syndrome.
- **Fasting may *reverse* type 2 diabetes**—In *Fast. Feast. Repeat.*, I talked about studies that had been conducted prior to 2019, all showing promise for those with type 2 diabetes. Since then, the news has only gotten better! In 2022, there was a new study published in *The Journal of Clinical Endocrinology & Metabolism* that found that 47.2 percent of participants who were part of the IF

intervention group "achieved diabetes remission" over a three-month intervention period. They also found: "After the 12-month follow-up, 44.4% (16/36) of the participants achieved sustained remission, with an HbA1c level of 6.33% (SD 0.87). The medication costs of the CMNT group were 77.22% lower than those of the control group (60.4/month vs 265.1/month)." WOW.

- **Fasting is anti-inflammatory**—You may already know that chronic inflammation has a serious negative impact on health, and IF lowers levels of inflammation within our bodies over time.

- **Fasting shows promise for those with autoimmune diseases**—Autoimmune diseases such as rheumatoid arthritis, psoriasis, multiple sclerosis, lupus, inflammatory bowel disease, and Hashimoto's thyroiditis are on the rise—particularly among women. Fasting can be beneficial in both preventing and controlling symptoms of many of these diseases.

- **Fasting has cardiovascular benefits**—Heart disease is considered to be the leading cause of death around the world. Fasting has been linked to reduced blood pressure, reduced resting heart rate, an improvement in the cardiovascular system's response to stress, and resistance of cardiac muscle to damage.

- **Fasting is excellent for brain health**—If we want to age well, we know we need to keep our brains healthy. Benefits of fasting include fewer signs of depression, improved memory, increased production of neurons, and an enhanced ability of our brains to ward off neurodegenerative diseases such as Alzheimer's and Parkinson's.

- **Fasting decreases visceral fat**—Increased levels of visceral fat—the fat found around your organs—have been linked to an increased risk of health conditions such as diabetes and even increased mortality. Intermittent fasting has been shown to lower both overall fat mass and this more dangerous visceral fat.

- **Fasting adjusts hunger and satiety hormones**—We are born with fully functioning appetite control signals. Think of a baby—a hungry baby cries until it is fed, and a baby that has had enough won't take one more drop. Somewhere along the way, however, we lose touch with these powerful signals. How does fasting help? Research shows that IF decreases ghrelin (the hunger hormone) and increases leptin (the satiety hormone). I'll talk more about this on day 17.

- **Fasting can "reset" the gut microbiome**—Over recent years, we have learned more and more about the importance of a healthy gut microbiome. We now know that our gut microbiomes are an important part of our immune systems' function and also play a key role in our overall metabolic health. Fasting has been shown to lead to reduced gut permeability, an increased diversity of the gut microbiome, and a shift to a gut population that is associated with leanness rather than obesity.

- **Fasting is antitumor and has positive effects during cancer treatment**—Fasting shows promise at both preventing tumor growth and also as a therapy that is useful as a part of a chemotherapy regimen. For anyone who has been or may be diagnosed with cancer, I recommend that you find an oncologist who is familiar with the research into using fasting along with chemotherapy.

- **Fasting increases autophagy**—You may be thinking:

What the heck is autophagy? I'll explain tomorrow, on day 5. Trust me! You want more of it.

EXTRA CREDIT READING
Chapter 2 of *Fast. Feast. Repeat.* The research supporting the health benefits of intermittent fasting is discussed and cited within that chapter.

DAILY INSPIRATION SPOTLIGHT:
Miki Earle, Sebago Lake, Maine
Intermittent Fasting Stories guest, episode 185

4

How long has she been an intermittent faster? *Between two and three years.*

My story is like that of so many women. With life and children and lifestyle, what was once a thin, healthy body became overweight (obese, actually) and emotionally uncomfortable. I had been successful as a business owner and life coach. It baffled me as to why I could not succeed at weight loss. Lord knows I had tried enough times in enough ways! In November of 2018, though I had sworn off ever dieting again, I made a commitment to myself that whatever it took, I was going to be at a healthy weight. My children and thirteen grandchildren deserved my being vital for all the days God allows me. After two months of the normal "dieting" attempts, I had lost some weight but was once again at a standstill. It was then that I "happened" to hear about The Obesity Code *and* Delay, Don't Deny. *I believe that was an answer to prayer. Everything I believed about losing weight was flipped on its head. I instinctively knew that what I* was learning about hormones and the body's ability to burn fat readily was true. I always believed that God had made our bodies to be health sustaining. But for the first time, I felt like I understood fully what that meant! Our bodies were not designed to be in perpetual intake mode. I needed it to complete the cycle of digestion and rest from digestion by fasting. So simple but so powerful! The rest of my journey, I managed my thoughts and emotions with all the coaching tools I knew so well, while living a consistent 18:6 fasting lifestyle. I cleaned up on the processed foods gradually but still enjoyed an occasional bagel and ice cream. I lost eighty pounds in nine months and truly experienced unimaginable freedom while losing weight. I remember the day that I looked at myself in the mirror and knew that this was the last time I would ever be overweight. I am a bit of an evangelist for things that improve a woman's life, so I found myself telling the whole world what I had discovered and soon moved my coaching business to include an online weight-loss coaching group, EverNu.net. There are now hundreds of women who have lost weight in our group using the same tools and knowledge that I gained in my own success. There is such freedom in this way of life!

ADVICE FROM MIKI

Adapting to a fasting lifestyle can be daunting at first, but with the gradual progression of increasing your clean fasting hours, you can get to your own sweet spot that produces steady weight loss as well as mental freedom. What we tell ourselves about what we must have to be happy is key to success in anything. I decided that whatever I did, I would do it with joy . . .

the hope and promise of good. Even at first, when I might feel deprived or limited, I would pull up the joy of the authority God has given us to be wise stewards of our lives. My saying no to something right now did not mean no forever. I lived in the expectation of success, and because of that, I got to experience that freedom and joy even in the struggles. There is a fasting lifestyle that will benefit each of us. Don't make the food the only focus in your weight loss. Immerse yourself in the good things of your life. Find creative outlets for expression of your presence in the world as you are changing your habits with food. Keep your commitment to yourself. The gift of your life is a treasure to be cherished.

4

**YOU HAVE ALL THE TOOLS YOU NEED TO SUCCEED.
ENJOY YOUR DAY! YOU'VE GOT THIS.**

HOW DID IT GO?
IT'S TIME TO REFLECT ON DAY 4.

TODAY (CHECK ALL THAT APPLY):

- ❏ I fasted clean (plain water, unflavored sparkling water, black unflavored coffee, plain tea)
- ❏ During the fast, I took time to reflect on the positive changes happening in my body
- ❏ Within my eating window, I ate until I was satisfied, and then I stopped
- ❏ I honored my "I've had enough" signals
- ❏ I stayed off the scale

FAST CHECK-IN

Rate the difficulty of today's fast on a scale from 1 to 10 (circle one):

1   2   3   4   5   6   7   8   9   **10**

(Today was easy! I sailed right through it.)   (Today was HARD! I struggled.)

During today's fast, I felt _____

_____

_____

_____

_____

_____

(*examples: exhilarated, hopeful, hungry, uncomfortable, bored, etc.*)

I used these strategies to manage my feelings today (check all that apply and add your own):

- ❏ I remembered my *why*
- ❏ I stayed busy
- ❏ I enjoyed a clean-fast-safe beverage
- ❏ I went on a walk
- ❏ I imagined my body tapping into my fat stores for fuel
- ❏ _____
  _____
- ❏ _____
  _____
- ❏ _____
  _____

EATING WINDOW CHECK-IN

Eating Window Length Goal: _____ **hours**
Actual Eating Window Length: _____ **hours**

How do I feel about today's eating window?

_____
_____
_____
_____
_____
_____
_____
_____
_____
_____

What went well? Was there anything that I struggled with during my eating window? _____

_____

_____

_____

_____

_____

_____

_____

_____

_____

_____

TODAY'S NSVS, OR NON-SCALE VICTORIES

One of the most powerful things we can do is acknowledge our Non-Scale Victories (NSVs). These can be physical (*pain reduction, better energy, mental clarity, etc.*) or emotional (*freedom around food, confidence, etc.*).

What were today's NSVs? _____

_____

_____

_____

_____

_____

_____

_____

_____

_____

REFLECTIONS

Today, I listened to my body when I: _____

_____

_____

_____

_____

_____

_____

_____

Today's *AHA!* moment(s): _____

_____

_____

_____

Something that is on my mind: _____

_____

_____

_____

_____

PREPARING FOR SUCCESS

Goal(s) and/or strategies for tomorrow: _____

_____

_____

_____

_____

_____

DAY 5: WHAT IS "AUTOPHAGY," AND WHY DO I WANT MORE OF IT?

Today's Date: _____

PLANNING FOR A SUCCESSFUL DAY 5

Today, I am following

- ❏ The *Easy Does It* Approach (twelve-hour window, low-carb ease-in breakfast and lunch, plus a regular dinner)
- ❏ The *Steady Build* Approach (eight-hour window, including lunch and dinner)
- ❏ The *Rip Off the Band-Aid* Approach (six-hour window, including lunch and dinner)

My personal goal(s) for today: _____

_____

_____

_____

_____

Daily Lesson from Gin: What is autophagy, and why do I want more of it?

What is autophagy? It literally means "self-eating." Autophagy is an important cellular mechanism that helps our cells survive when faced with stressors, including times of starvation. *Starvation* is a harsh word, and when we are intermittent fasters, it's important to be clear that we aren't starving ourselves. We fast, and then we **feast**. We intentionally include periods of the day where we fast clean, which is different from times of famine when our bodies are in danger.

Increased autophagy is one of the most powerful benefits of the clean fast, and it's one of my favorites. Once you understand what autophagy does within our bodies, I think you'll agree.

To understand autophagy, think of it as our bodies' ultimate upcycling program. What is upcycling? According to Wikipedia, upcycling "*is the process of transforming by-products, waste materials, useless, or unwanted products into new materials or products of better quality and environmental value.*" That is precisely what autophagy does: autophagy transforms our bodies' *by-products, waste materials, useless, or unwanted products* into *new materials or products of better quality and environmental value*!

I'm going to include an analogy I first wrote about in *Fast. Feast. Repeat.*, because I haven't thought of a better way to explain it. (Teachers know repetition is how we learn, so when you read this again in *Fast. Feast. Repeat.*, it will sink in even better the second time around.)

As you may know, I was a teacher for twenty-eight years. Elementary school teachers are *great* upcyclers! Somehow, we teachers are all born with the instinct to take junk and turn it into something useful. We can make comfy seating nooks out of old tires, discarded paint buckets, and milk crates we ~~stole~~ borrowed from the cafeteria. Give us your old cereal boxes and we can make board games, playing cards, and book display shelves. Just as teachers are born with the upcycling instinct, so are our bodies. Trash becomes treasure, whether we are upcycling in our classrooms or upcycling within our own bodies.

So, our bodies use the process of autophagy to recycle damaged or unwanted cell parts to use them for energy or for building blocks for new growth. Damaged organelles? Autophagy upcycles their parts! Intracellular pathogens? Autophagy to the rescue! Got cellular junk? Autophagy for the win!

When we are fasting, autophagy increases to ensure our survival in the absence of food intake.

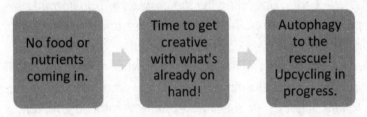

I absolutely love the thought that while I am fasting every day, my body is looking for old cellular junk to remake into a spiffy new body part.

Our goal is to ensure that autophagy is allowed to occur on a frequent basis, just as nature intended. When autophagy is blocked somehow within the body, this can lead to the onset of cancer, liver disease, accelerated aging, metabolic syndrome, or neurodegeneration. I want to make sure that I am experiencing all the benefits of increased autophagy on a daily basis.

This can cause a lot of confusion. When does autophagy happen, exactly? How can we *know* it's happening? Will we experience increased autophagy when we follow a daily intermittent fasting approach, or do we need to do extended fasts to reap these benefits?

Think about this for a minute. Would your body have an amazing cellular cleaning process that required you to fast for days and days to access it? It doesn't make any sense, does it?

Our bodies are designed to be metabolically flexible. Before the modern era, our ancestors had to hunt and gather to be fed, so they would have periods of time where they were naturally in the fasted state. They relied on ketosis to fuel their brains, giving them the mental clarity and energy to go out and find the food they needed. This metabolic flexibility would have gotten them through both the daily quest for food and the lean times.

Increased autophagy is part of this important adaptation and is linked to the state of ketosis. Both of these processes happen when your metabolic switch is flipped and your body has to scrounge around for fuel. Think about it like this: imagine that you haven't been to the grocery store for a long time, you're snowed in, and your fridge and pantry are fairly bare . . . but you're hungry! You will need to dig around to see what you have lying around that you could make into a meal. This is what happens when your body is in the fasted state: your body is foraging around within for fuel (which leads to *fat burning and ketosis*) and also searching for whatever building blocks can be torn down and reused (which happens through increased *autophagy*). So, while ketosis and autophagy are *not* the same process, they both occur when the body has a need to scrounge around to see what's on hand.

You'll often hear someone in the intermittent fasting community say that autophagy doesn't ramp up until someone is twenty-four to thirty-six hours into the fasted state. That statement causes a lot of confusion for many people, and that's because it doesn't tell the whole story! I'll tell you more about this on day 9, when I teach you how we get into ketosis once we deplete our liver glycogen sufficiently to get into the fat-burning state. It's true that it might take someone twenty-four to thirty-six hours to do this (or even longer) *if they are beginning with full glycogen stores*. But—and this is important—after our bodies become metabolically flexible, we no longer start each day with full glycogen stores! I'll teach you about becoming metabolically flexible on day 9, so stay tuned.

The takeaway is this: we are able to get into ketosis daily when we are in the fasted state (*this may happen at around hour twelve of the fast, though it might take as long as sixteen to twenty-plus hours, depending on what and how much you eat, your activity level, and even how much insulin your body has circulating*). And, since we know that when ketosis ramps up, so does autophagy, you can be assured that you are receiving benefits from increased autophagy without having to fast regularly for twenty-four to thirty-six hours or beyond.

It's true that if you fast longer you'll get more deeply into ketosis and experience even higher levels of autophagy, but it is not required. Trust that your body will make the most of your daily fasting period, with no longer fasts required . . . unless you *want* to fast longer.

For now, simply be confident that your body has all the tools it needs to do what it needs to do behind the scenes, and that includes increased autophagy.

DAILY INSPIRATION SPOTLIGHT:
Jana Dworetzky, Thornhill, Ontario, Canada
Intermittent Fasting Stories guest, episode 171

How long has she been an intermittent faster? *Between two and three years.*

Before I started IF, I weighed 240 pounds. I was on two different types of injectable medication for inflammatory arthritis that I was diagnosed with at age thirteen months. I had just been told that I had NAFLD (nonalcoholic fatty liver disease), and I knew that a diagnosis of diabetes was just around the corner. I was facing a lifetime of health ailments as I entered my forties. My daughter, who was seven years old at the time, couldn't wrap her arms around me when she hugged me. It brought tears to my eyes. I knew I had to do something and that a lifestyle change was in order. I had tried every conventional diet under the sun throughout my entire life, starting from the time I was in grade 6. One week after a friend first mentioned the phrase intermittent fasting *to me, a second friend mentioned it. It felt as if the universe was trying to tell me something. At first, I felt that this was not for me—I couldn't do it, I loved breakfast too much, and black coffee? Never. Yet something I had never heard of previously was starting to be trending in my life. I started the very next day, cold turkey, and I haven't looked back since. My health improved within weeks. My NAFLD was reversed within the first month of IF. I have since come off all injectable medication for arthritis and have never had a flare-up since. My inflammation markers consistently are normal. My average blood sugar levels are 5.9, and I have no concerns about becoming a diabetic. To date, I have lost a*

5

little over eighty pounds. I lost the weight within the first year and a half of my IF lifestyle and have maintained for the next year and a half as I approach my three-year fast-iversary. While I have not lost more scale weight, my body has continued to change. I hear regularly from people I see often that I look like I have lost even more weight. Scale-wise, I know this isn't the truth, yet my body continues to evolve. [Note from Gin: This is body recomposition in action! As you lose fat and maintain or build muscle, you shrink in size, but the scale may not reflect those changes.] My health continues to improve. I have always known that to be successful in weight loss, I'd have to change my lifestyle, and diets have never stuck. IF is the first time in my life where I have made the sustainable changes neces- sary to never worry that I'm going to become obese again. I'm happy with what I've accomplished and thrilled to be in this healthy body. After all, I keep telling my husband now that I'm going to live forever, and I can't wait to enjoy my life as I do so.

ADVICE FROM JANA

To the new IFers, it's true that this lifestyle is hard in contemplation and easy in execution. It's not as hard as you think it's going to be. To those restarting IF, IF is always there when you're ready. This lifestyle is adaptable and needs to work with your life in order to be the sustainable lifestyle change it needs to be. As Gin says, "Tweak it till it's easy." You just have to try different pathways to find the one that works for you. I believe that knowledge is power, and if you under- stand why something works, it will just make sense.

**YOU HAVE ALL THE TOOLS YOU NEED TO SUCCEED.
ENJOY YOUR DAY! YOU'VE GOT THIS.**

HOW DID IT GO?
IT'S TIME TO REFLECT ON DAY 5.

TODAY (CHECK ALL THAT APPLY):

❏ I fasted clean (plain water, unflavored sparkling water, black unflavored coffee, plain tea)
❏ During the fast, I took time to reflect on the positive changes happening in my body
❏ Within my eating window, I ate until I was satisfied, and then I stopped
❏ I honored my "I've had enough" signals
❏ I stayed off the scale

FAST CHECK-IN

Rate the difficulty of today's fast on a scale from 1 to 10 (circle one):

1 2 3 4 5 6 7 8 9 **10**

(Today was easy! I sailed right through it.)   (Today was HARD! I struggled.)

During today's fast, I felt _____
_____
_____
_____
_____
_____

(*examples: exhilarated, hopeful, hungry, uncomfortable, bored, etc.*)

I used these strategies to manage my feelings today (check all that apply and add your own):

- ❏ I remembered my *why*
- ❏ I stayed busy
- ❏ I enjoyed a clean-fast-safe beverage
- ❏ I went on a walk
- ❏ I imagined my body tapping into my fat stores for fuel
- ❏ _____
  _____
- ❏ _____
  _____
- ❏ _____
  _____

EATING WINDOW CHECK-IN

Eating Window Length Goal: _____ hours
Actual Eating Window Length: _____ hours

How do I feel about today's eating window?

_____
_____
_____
_____
_____
_____
_____
_____
_____

What went well? Was there anything that I struggled with during my eating window? _____

_____

_____

_____

_____

_____

_____

_____

_____

_____

TODAY'S NSVS, OR NON-SCALE VICTORIES

One of the most powerful things we can do is acknowledge our Non-Scale Victories (NSVs). These can be physical (*pain reduction, better energy, mental clarity, etc.*) or emotional (*freedom around food, confidence, etc.*).

What were today's NSVs? _____

_____

_____

_____

_____

_____

_____

_____

_____

REFLECTIONS

Today, I listened to my body when I: _____

_____

_____

_____

_____

_____

_____

_____

Today's *AHA!* moment(s): _____

_____

_____

_____

Something that is on my mind: _____

_____

_____

_____

PREPARING FOR SUCCESS

Goal(s) and/or strategies for tomorrow: _____

_____

_____

_____

_____

DAY 6: FOOD, GLORIOUS FOOD!
EAT WHATEVER *YOU* WANT

Today's Date: _____

PLANNING FOR A SUCCESSFUL DAY 6

Today, I am following

- ❏ The *Easy Does It* Approach (twelve-hour window, low-carb ease-in breakfast and lunch, plus a regular dinner)
- ❏ The *Steady Build* Approach (eight-hour window, including lunch and dinner)
- ❏ The *Rip Off the Band-Aid* Approach (six-hour window, including lunch and dinner)

My personal goal(s) for today: _____

_____

_____

_____

_____

Daily Lesson from Gin: Food, glorious food! Eat whatever YOU want.

When you begin an intermittent fasting lifestyle, you may be drawn to the concept of eating "whatever you want." You may be like I was when I first began IF in 2014—I was diet-weary from years of following restrictive eating plans. I wanted to simply have the freedom to eat food with no angst.

So, when I started IF, my "diet" could best be described as "eating like a college freshman who has been let loose in the dining hall for the first time." I embraced the "eat whatever you want" mindset fully.

A funny thing happened along the way, however. The freedom to eat *whatever I wanted* gave me space to figure out over time what I really DID want to eat.

It turns out: I don't really want to eat junk foods. Giving myself permission to eat whatever I wanted taught me what I really *did* want to eat. This process took years, but the way I eat in 2023 is very different from the way I ate in 2014, and it happened naturally without me forcing it.

I'm serious when I tell you that a great deal of freedom comes from learning to eat whatever you want.

Not many phrases lead to such confusion as *eat whatever you want*, however. Let's talk about what it means and what it doesn't mean.

When you live an intermittent fasting lifestyle, you can truly "eat whatever *you* want." But you can't "EAT ***WHATEVER*** YOU WANT!"

Wait a minute, Gin . . . Aren't those the exact same words? Well, yes, but also NO. Not even close.

Let me explain.

The difference is in the emphasis. You get to decide how you want to eat. You get to eat whatever works for **YOU**. Whatever **YOU** want.

On the other hand, if you "EAT ***WHATEVER*** YOU WANT!" and what you "want" is nothing but fast food, potato chips, and Pop-Tarts, you probably won't feel great. When you feel gross after eating those types of foods, you learn that you don't want to keep feeling that way. Wanting to feel better is a powerful motivator.

One of the best parts of living an IF lifestyle is how it nudges you toward making decisions that make you feel great.

When you used to eat all day long, you probably got used to how you felt. Maybe you were sluggish, and you may have had aches and pains or brain fog. That was your "normal," and you didn't even realize how bad you felt.

As you continue down the IF path, however, you're going to start to feel better and better over time. Once your body is fat adapted (which I'll explain on day 9), you'll feel amazing during your daily fast. Once you open your window, if you choose foods that make you feel gross, you'll notice it a lot more than you would've in your eating-all-day past.

As I mentioned already, wanting to feel better is a powerful motivator.

Here's an example of that from my life. In the years that I've been an IFer, I've realized that most fried foods (especially if the restaurant isn't great at changing their frying oil) make my stomach hurt. Do I enjoy the feeling of a stomachache? Of course not. So, I make choices to avoid having a stomachache. I don't do it because some diet book told me "fried foods are bad." I do it because my *body* told me.

Powerful difference.

I can eat all the fried foods I want to eat. I **always** get to eat whatever *I* want. But because I don't want a stomachache, I *don't want to eat cheap fried foods*.

My goal is for you to feel empowered to choose the foods that work best for your body. I'm not going to tell you that the only way to succeed is to follow a keto or low-carb diet, or that you must become a vegan, or that you can never have fried foods or sugar again.

That being said, maybe your body *does* feel best with fewer carbs, or maybe you're the opposite and you're someone who thrives on a high-carb, plant-based diet. Maybe you feel best when you eat a lot of meat, but maybe you feel better when you don't eat meat at all. Maybe fried foods make *you* feel gross, like they do for me.

The truth is—there are a zillion ways you might choose to eat, and what works best for *your* body isn't necessarily what will work best for *my* body. This is due to bio-individuality, a big word that simply means that we are all biologically unique. It has to do with all the things that make you YOU, from your genetics to the diverse residents of your gut microbiome.

I genuinely believe that you could follow me around all day and eat exactly what I eat and have different results. Our bodies aren't the same.

So, it wouldn't make any sense for me to tell you *what* to eat.

This doesn't mean that all foods are created equal. You'll understand that ultra-processed foods, such as packaged snacks, sodas, and other chemical-filled concoctions, aren't even really *food* once you understand how the body works. A Dorito might taste delicious, but it won't nourish your body. I'm sure you've heard the words *empty calories* before. That's what I am talking about here.

The ONE thing all the health-focused experts seem to agree on these days—whether they are promoting a keto diet, a vegan lifestyle, the Paleo diet, or any other healthy way of eating—is that REAL FOOD is going to be superior to ultra-processed foods, every time. I've never seen a nutritional study that found health benefits associated with a ~~crappy~~ low-quality, ultra-processed diet.

In summary: eat whatever **you** want. Throughout this process, YOU are empowered to decide what foods you choose to include in your daily eating window.

But don't think that you can **EAT WHATEVER YOU WANT!** and expect to feel your best. Real food is delicious and satisfying, and every time you choose real food over ultra-processed foods, you're making a great choice for your body.

If foods make you feel bad after you eat them, those foods aren't worth eating frequently.

Over time, you'll learn to trust yourself. Eating shouldn't involve complicated math formulas or food plans. Choose foods that are delicious and that make you feel great after you eat them. We call those foods *window-worthy*. When I open my window, I am not going to waste it on subpar food. I want to have something that is delicious, and I want to feel great after I eat.

That doesn't mean I aim for dietary perfection. While I know the humble Dorito is totally fake food, I can choose to include whatever I want to eat within my window.

If I ate a bag of Doritos, I would feel awful. If I have a few Doritos after a nutritious meal that satisfies my body, I feel just fine, and I don't have any guilt about it.

Nobody tells me what to eat or what not to eat. I get to decide.

And so do you.

After reading this section, you may think that you have to "clean up" what you are eating immediately. That's NOT what I want you to take away from this section.

Instead, please don't make any radical changes to how you're eating just yet. Here's why: your body is learning how to do something new right now. If you also try to change everything that you're eating, you're more likely to crash and burn. So, don't try to make too many changes all at once.

As you make your way through the rest of your FAST Start, I don't want you to stress about what you're eating. Instead, approach each day as a learning experience. Figure out what makes you feel great and what doesn't. No judgment, just curiosity and an open mind.

EXTRA CREDIT READING
Chapter 14 of *Fast. Feast. Repeat.* for a discussion of bio-individuality, and chapter 17 for information about the importance of prioritizing real food over ultra-processed foods.

DAILY INSPIRATION SPOTLIGHT:
Melinda Spangenberg, Concord, North Carolina
Intermittent Fasting Stories guest, episode 276

How long has she been an intermittent faster? *Between three and four years.*

My decision to begin intermittent fasting occurred shortly after my mother was diagnosed with dementia. I began IF for purely health-related reasons; the weight loss, which was very much needed (seventy-plus pounds), was a surprise benefit. About eighteen months into my journey, my father had a major stroke. I could feel like the deck is stacked against me, but I choose to acknowledge the genetic health challenges and fight back with IF. I truly believe that this is the best lifestyle to alter what used to be considered inevitable. Of course, there are no guarantees, and without a crystal ball, I can't predict what twists and turns my health will take. What I do know is that with IF, I am living my best life now, and going forward, I expect that to continue. My interview was recorded just prior to the American Thanksgiving holiday, which segues into the December holiday season, which in 2022 happened to include my son's wedding. There were a lot of events happening that included food and drink. Even without the wedding, this time of year has always been difficult for me, and I still find that somewhat true even as I enter my fourth year of fasting and over two years in my goal range. Learning to listen to my body and follow the signals it sends me is an evolving process. As a sixty-two-year-old woman, I've learned that my body will guide me, but I must be willing to listen and learn. Some things that I could eat and drink at a younger age no longer serve me, so I make a choice to not partake of those things. Because it is my choice, I don't feel deprived, and I feel healthier in the long run. I will admit I gained a few pounds this last season, and that's okay. When I returned to my normal fasting schedule and healthy food choices, the weight returned to its normal place. Life is not static, and neither is my weight.

6

ADVICE FROM MELINDA

If you are a new intermittent faster or someone who is restarting, my advice would be to determine both your why *and* what *for intermittent fasting. Ask yourself how you would like to feel in one year, five years, ten years, twenty years, and whether IF would be beneficial to attaining your long-term goals. Life is not linear; give yourself grace to move through the different seasons, knowing that with IF as your touchstone you will be able to live your best life season after season.*

**YOU HAVE ALL THE TOOLS YOU NEED TO SUCCEED.
ENJOY YOUR DAY! YOU'VE GOT THIS.**

HOW DID IT GO?
IT'S TIME TO REFLECT ON DAY 6.

TODAY (CHECK ALL THAT APPLY):

- ❏ I fasted clean (plain water, unflavored sparkling water, black unflavored coffee, plain tea)
- ❏ During the fast, I took time to reflect on the positive changes happening in my body
- ❏ Within my eating window, I ate until I was satisfied, and then I stopped
- ❏ I honored my "I've had enough" signals
- ❏ I stayed off the scale

FAST CHECK-IN

Rate the difficulty of today's fast on a scale from 1 to 10 (circle one):

1 2 3 4 5 6 7 8 9 **10**

(Today was easy! I sailed right through it.)   (Today was HARD! I struggled.)

During today's fast, I felt _____

_____

_____

_____

_____

_____

(*examples: exhilarated, hopeful, hungry, uncomfortable, bored, etc.*)

I used these strategies to manage my feelings today (check all that apply and add your own):

- ❏ I remembered my *why*
- ❏ I stayed busy
- ❏ I enjoyed a clean-fast-safe beverage
- ❏ I went on a walk
- ❏ I imagined my body tapping into my fat stores for fuel
- ❏ _____
  _____
- ❏ _____
  _____
- ❏ _____
  _____

EATING WINDOW CHECK-IN

Eating Window Length Goal: _____ hours
Actual Eating Window Length: _____ hours

How do I feel about today's eating window?

_____
_____
_____
_____
_____
_____
_____
_____
_____
_____

What went well? Was there anything that I struggled with during my eating window? _____

_____

_____

_____

_____

_____

_____

_____

_____

_____

TODAY'S NSVS, OR NON-SCALE VICTORIES

One of the most powerful things we can do is acknowledge our Non-Scale Victories (NSVs). These can be physical (*pain reduction, better energy, mental clarity, etc.*) or emotional (*freedom around food, confidence, etc.*).

What were today's NSVs? _____

_____

_____

_____

_____

_____

_____

_____

_____

REFLECTIONS

Today, I listened to my body when I: _____
_____
_____
_____
_____
_____
_____
_____
_____

Today's *AHA!* moment(s): _____
_____
_____
_____
_____

Something that is on my mind: _____
_____
_____
_____
_____

PREPARING FOR SUCCESS

Goal(s) and/or strategies for tomorrow: _____
_____
_____
_____
_____
_____

DAY 7: SATURDAY IS NOT A SPECIAL OCCASION; IT HAPPENS EVERY WEEK

Today's Date: _____

PLANNING FOR A SUCCESSFUL DAY 7

Today, I am following

- ❑ The *Easy Does It* Approach (twelve-hour window, low-carb ease-in breakfast and lunch, plus a regular dinner)
- ❑ The *Steady Build* Approach (eight-hour window, including lunch and dinner)
- ❑ The *Rip Off the Band-Aid* Approach (six-hour window, including lunch and dinner)

My personal goal(s) for today: _____

_____

_____

_____

_____

_____

7

Daily Lesson from Gin: Saturday is not a special occasion: it happens every week.

If you've read my first book, *Delay, Don't Deny*, you may remember that I have a chapter with the same title as today's daily lesson in that book. I didn't mention it explicitly in *Fast. Feast. Repeat.*, which I think was a mistake. So, I am talking about it here, within the first week of your FAST Start, and that's by design.

You see, the *"weekends are a special occasion"* mindset trips up a lot of intermittent fasters, and I think it is really important to proactively decide how you're going to handle weekends and other celebratory events that pop up.

If you're a *Seinfeld* fan like I am, perhaps you've seen the episode where Elaine's office has frequent and multiple celebrations for every occasion you can imagine. The episode "The Frogger" ends with Elaine eating a vintage wedding cake that her boss, Peterman, bought at auction for $29,000. All did not end well for Elaine's digestive system that day, since the cake was decades old.

While *Seinfeld* is a comedy, watching that episode reminds me of what it's like for many of us to go into the workplace daily. I was an elementary school teacher for twenty-eight years, and someone was always celebrating something. On a daily basis, you could usually find cupcakes or some other kind of "treats" in the teachers' workroom. Many (if not most) places of work are like that, too.

Over time, I realized that grocery store cupcakes sitting out in the workroom were not actually special, and they were definitely not worth breaking my fast for. So, if I wanted to have something that was sitting around, I learned how to delay it . . . I would pack it up in a ziplock bag and take it home for later.

Most of the time, however, those treats were *not* window-worthy. It got a lot easier to see them sitting there and not want one at all . . . now *or* later. That didn't happen on day 1, or even in the first few months. It took a while for me to get there, but I am now at the place where I wouldn't eat a grocery store cupcake for any reason. (A high-quality and delicious cupcake? That is another story entirely!)

Even after I had mastered the avoidance of the minefield of celebratory treats that surrounded me daily, I still struggled with one type of special occasion mindset, and that was *the weekend*.

Remember the song "Working for the Weekend"? That was my mantra. And in an elementary school, weekends started on Friday. We could wear *jeans*. Every Friday felt like a celebration. The problem was . . . so did Saturday and Sunday.

Then Monday would roll around. Back to work. And the cycle continued, week after week. Any positive progress I made from Monday to Thursday was undone from Friday to Sunday.

Even for people who don't practice intermittent fasting, the "weekends are a special occasion" mentality can be a problem. Treating every weekend like one big food-and-drink party isn't a great strategy for anyone. How many people "start over" on their "diets" every Monday?

Don't let that be you.

During the FAST Start, you want to nail the clean fast every day, including the weekend. If a true special occasion pops up, such as your birthday or Christmas, you can shift your eating window to accommodate any celebration that involves food. Maybe you have a ten-hour eating window for that one day only, and the next day, you're back to the FAST Start eating window length you've chosen. One day won't ruin anything.

But treating every Saturday like it's a special occasion? That makes it a lot harder for your body to adjust to fasting

7

and delays you becoming fat adapted. (I'll tell you more about that on day 9 . . . but you definitely don't want to delay the fat-adaptation process if you can help it.)

One other sticky situation you may find popping up has to do with the expectations of others. Maybe *you* are determined, but someone else is pressuring you to eat.

Think of what tools you can add to your toolbox when other people may expect you to join them in an eating experience. Here are a few:

"Thank you! I'll save that for later!" is always appropriate. You never have to eat something in front of others just to please them.

"Instead of meeting for breakfast, could we meet for lunch?" works beautifully. Or you could meet for breakfast and just drink black coffee. It's not weird. Lots of people do that.

"I'm not hungry right now." It is always your right to not be hungry. It's also no one's business why you are or aren't eating.

"I already ate." I only use this one when my eating window is closed for the day. Even though I already mentioned that it's no one's business if and when you eat, I don't like to lie. I only tell people I already ate if that is true.

Some people really won't take no for an answer, and I think that is really rude. Think about it this way: if you had a life-threatening shellfish allergy, would you eat shrimp just because everyone else is eating it? Of course you wouldn't.

It is your *right* to choose what you put into your body and when. Anyone who is upset because you don't want to have what they are having has deeper issues that are not your problem . . . Don't make their issues into *your* issues.

DAILY INSPIRATION SPOTLIGHT:
Patrice Hegel, Howell, New Jersey
Intermittent Fasting Stories guest, episode 235

How long has she been an intermittent faster? *Between two and three years.*

I was a skinny kid, but put on weight as I entered my forties and fifties. Over those years, I tried some different diet plans: WeightWatchers (where I'd felt deprived and hungry), Nutrisystem (where the food tasted artificial), and even a doctor-directed plan that included medication. Each worked for a while, but not without a lot of hunger, and they were not sustainable. Once I'd stop the diet, I'd gain back the weight and a bit more . . . probably messing up my metabolism in the process. January of 2020, I saw a photo of myself and how much weight I'd gained after menopause. I'm five foot five, and at that time, I was about to turn sixty and weighed 197 pounds. I again tried WeightWatchers and was sad and hungry. I heard about intermittent fasting from a friend and started researching. I came upon Delay, Don't Deny and decided to try it. I embraced the clean fast. When the pandemic happened that March, I went all in, because here was something I could control when so much of our world felt out of control. I gradually worked my way to OMAD (one meal a day), and my sweet spot now is usually between twenty- and twenty-two-hour fasts. For a couple of months in the beginning, I'd put a piece of Himalayan sea salt under my tongue (because minerals don't break a fast), but that backfired and made me hungry. Once I stopped that, fasting became so much easier. Over the next two and a half years, I slowly lost weight and improved my health. The weight came off in ways it never had before. I was patient because I knew that internally good things were happening along with the weight loss. Ultimately, I lost sixty-two pounds. My inflammation went away, my blood test results all improved, my energy increased, I became sharper mentally and continue to work in the fasted state. People started asking me what I was doing . . . including my doctors, one of whom then started fasting as well! Since then, I've been able to maintain within a five-pound weight range. I've learned to listen to my body and can now recognize real hunger and satiety. This has become my way of life. On special occasions, I'll open my window early and enjoy without guilt. Diet brain is gone. There's no falling off the wagon, because there no longer is a wagon! I like my body, am at peace with my weight, and happily advocate for anyone who's interested and wants to explore fasting. I'm proof postmenopausal women can lose weight and keep it off!

ADVICE FROM PATRICE

The clean fast is so important because it helps in managing hunger; things get so much easier when that's mastered. Have patience . . . I was a turtle, but my body continued to change and drop weight gradually over two and a half years, getting me back to the weight I was comfortable with in my thirties. Educate yourself about the science behind the process and the benefits to your body besides the weight loss. This truly is the health plan with the benefit of weight loss.

YOU HAVE ALL THE TOOLS YOU NEED TO SUCCEED.
ENJOY YOUR DAY! YOU'VE GOT THIS.

HOW DID IT GO?
IT'S TIME TO REFLECT ON DAY 7.

TODAY (CHECK ALL THAT APPLY):

- ❏ I fasted clean (plain water, unflavored sparkling water, black unflavored coffee, plain tea)
- ❏ During the fast, I took time to reflect on the positive changes happening in my body
- ❏ Within my eating window, I ate until I was satisfied, and then I stopped
- ❏ I honored my "I've had enough" signals
- ❏ I stayed off the scale

FAST CHECK-IN

Rate the difficulty of today's fast on a scale from 1 to 10 (circle one):

1　2　3　4　5　6　7　8　9　**10**

(Today was easy! I sailed right through it.)　　　　(Today was HARD! I struggled.)

During today's fast, I felt _____

_____

_____

_____

_____

_____

(*examples: exhilarated, hopeful, hungry, uncomfortable, bored, etc.*)

I used these strategies to manage my feelings today (check all that apply and add your own):

- ❏ I remembered my *why*
- ❏ I stayed busy
- ❏ I enjoyed a clean-fast-safe beverage
- ❏ I went on a walk
- ❏ I imagined my body tapping into my fat stores for fuel
- ❏ _____
  _____
- ❏ _____
  _____
- ❏ _____
  _____

EATING WINDOW CHECK-IN

Eating Window Length Goal: _____ hours
Actual Eating Window Length: _____ hours

How do I feel about today's eating window?

_____
_____
_____
_____
_____
_____
_____
_____
_____
_____

What went well? Was there anything that I struggled with during my eating window? _____

_____

_____

_____

_____

_____

_____

_____

_____

_____

TODAY'S NSVS, OR NON-SCALE VICTORIES

One of the most powerful things we can do is acknowledge our Non-Scale Victories (NSVs). These can be physical (*pain reduction, better energy, mental clarity, etc.*) or emotional (*freedom around food, confidence, etc.*).

What were today's NSVs? _____

_____

_____

_____

_____

_____

_____

_____

_____

_____

REFLECTIONS

Today, I listened to my body when I: _____

_____

_____

_____

_____

_____

_____

_____

Today's *AHA!* moment(s): _____

_____

_____

_____

Something that is on my mind: _____

_____

_____

_____

PREPARING FOR SUCCESS

Goal(s) and/or strategies for tomorrow: _____

_____

_____

_____

_____

WEEK 2 PLAN

Which approach did you choose last week?

- ☐ The *Easy Does It* Approach (twelve-hour window, low-carb ease-in breakfast and lunch, plus a regular dinner)
- ☐ The *Steady Build* Approach (eight-hour window, including lunch and dinner)
- ☐ The *Rip Off the Band-Aid* Approach (six-hour window, including lunch and dinner)

How did it go?
- ☐ It was too easy! I think I can ramp it up this week.
- ☐ It was JUST RIGHT. Not too hard, not too easy.
- ☐ It was too much for me. I am going to scale it back this week.

Which approach will you follow for week 2?
- ☐ The *Easy Does It* Approach (ten-hour window, low-carb ease-in breakfast or early lunch, low-carb ease-in snack, plus a regular dinner)
- ☐ The *Steady Build* Approach (seven-hour window, including lunch and dinner)
- ☐ The *Rip Off the Band-Aid* Approach (six-hour window, including lunch *or* snack, and dinner)

DAY 8: *TWEAK IT TILL IT'S EASY* DURING THE FAST START

Today's Date: _____

PLANNING FOR A SUCCESSFUL DAY 8

Today, I am following

- ❏ The *Easy Does It* Approach (ten-hour window, low-carb ease-in breakfast or early lunch, low-carb ease-in snack, plus a regular dinner)
- ❏ The *Steady Build* Approach (seven-hour window, including lunch and dinner)
- ❏ The *Rip Off the Band-Aid* Approach (six-hour window, including lunch *or* snack, and dinner)

My personal goal(s) for today: _____

_____

_____

_____

_____

8

Daily Lesson from Gin: Tweak it till it's easy during the FAST Start.

Congratulations on completing the first week of your FAST Start! By doing that, you are well on your way. All you have to do is keep doing it, day by day.

I want to teach you one of our most important mantras: "Tweak it till it's easy."

In our community, we often say those words:

"Tweak it till it's easy."

And that is exactly what we mean.

As you continue through the FAST Start, not every moment will be easy. That is *not* what I mean.

Don't expect it to be easy *every moment*. We tweak it **till** it's easy. Easy is the ultimate goal.

You won't be at "easy" immediately. But every day shouldn't be a terrible struggle, either. We shouldn't have to force it to the point that we feel awful.

As you planned how you're going to approach week 2, you may have decided you want to ramp things up. There's nothing wrong with ramping up if you feel ready to do so.

But don't force it if you aren't ready. Part of tweaking it till it's easy is making sure you aren't doing more than your body is ready for. There is never anything wrong with scaling it back if you need to.

What are some things you can do this week to tweak it till it's easy?

- **Play with your window timing**—It's fine to shift your daily eating window around. As an example, if you're aiming for a seven-hour window this week, you could try noon–7:00 p.m. one day, and 10:00 a.m.–5:00 p.m. the next. As long as you stick to the seven-hour boundary, your window was a success.
- **Stay busy**—When I was learning how to cement my daily eating window habit, I would often plan to run errands

in the last couple of hours before my window opened. When I was out and about, it was easier to delay opening my window than when I was only steps from the fridge and pantry.

- **Plan for eating window success**—Have a plan for how you will open your eating window. That can prevent the experience of wandering around the kitchen eating anything you can find.
- **Focus on foods that satisfy your body**—While you always get to eat what *you* want, some foods are going to be better choices than others. Our bodies are searching for nutrients, and whenever you can choose high-quality real foods over ultra-processed foods, your body is going to be more satisfied. I don't want you to think of foods as "good" or "bad" but instead think of foods as "satisfying" or "unsatisfying." As an example, if I opened my window with a bag of potato chips, I wouldn't be very satisfied. A huge loaded baked potato, however? I would feel extremely satisfied after eating that.

DAILY INSPIRATION SPOTLIGHT:
Melissa Denny, Brighton, Colorado
Intermittent Fasting Stories guest, episode 151

8

How long has she been an intermittent faster? *Between three and four years.*

My IF journey started about a year after the birth of my second child in August 2019. I had used calories in / calories out in the past to lose weight and had stuck with it religiously for a year. It worked for a little while, until it didn't. I kept reducing the number of calories I was consuming, increased the intensity of my workouts, and the scale started to climb back up. I knew of some friends trying intermittent fasting, and one of them added me to a Delay, Don't Deny group on Facebook. I lurked in the group for a while, unsure that I would ever be able to skip a meal, being a three-meals-a-day and two-snacks girl for quite some time. I went on a vacation, and when I saw the photos, it was my aha moment. I had to do something drastic, so I started fasting with a 16:8 protocol the next day. I found immediate success, losing thirteen pounds in the first month and feeling incredible. I checked the group several times a day and even got the courage to post a couple of before-and-after photos. People were so encouraging and supportive. The positive feedback I got from others kept me going, and I spent time each day encouraging others and answering questions in the group. As my fasting muscles grew, I did longer fasts, tried out some Meal-less Mondays and loved them! [Note from Gin: To learn more about Meal-less Mondays and other alternate-day fasting approaches, read the ADF chapter of Fast. Feast. Repeat.] I settled on somewhere between an 18:6 and 20:4 with ADF down days mixed in and lost another thirty-five pounds, bringing my total to just under fifty pounds lost. I continued to engage with the groups and found myself as one of the admins of a spin-off group that has grown to over twelve thousand members! I follow a plant-based diet, and I am a runner, but I was those things before IF. Intermittent fasting has just elevated those things. I do the large majority of all my runs and workouts fasted. I have improved my paces and won age group awards in races all since starting IF. I like to keep my body guessing and don't really follow a set *routine. Most of my weeks look like Meal-less Monday, up day on Tuesday, 20:4 on Wednesday and Thursday, and then 18:6 for the weekend. This works for me, and I am able to effortlessly maintain my weight. My body continues to change as body recomposition does its thing. IF gives me a quiet confidence and keeps me feeling healthy and strong in my body. It feels so routine now and is a lifestyle I will never give up!*

ADVICE FROM MELISSA

My advice is to find community. I feel like the IF community has been such a huge part of my journey. I learn so much from others and get so much joy in leading others to the IF lifestyle and helping them along the way by answering questions and hosting challenges in my Facebook group. So many people have encouraged me, and I would not be where I am without their support. If you lost your way, go back to the community. Join a group, listen to a podcast, or read another book about IF. All these things will help you to be surrounded by positive influences that will support you back onto the right path and pick you up when you fall, just like others have done for me along the way.

8

**YOU HAVE ALL THE TOOLS YOU NEED TO SUCCEED.
ENJOY YOUR DAY! YOU'VE GOT THIS.**

HOW DID IT GO?
IT'S TIME TO REFLECT ON DAY 8.

TODAY (CHECK ALL THAT APPLY):

- ❏ I fasted clean (plain water, unflavored sparkling water, black unflavored coffee, plain tea)
- ❏ During the fast, I took time to reflect on the positive changes happening in my body
- ❏ Within my eating window, I ate until I was satisfied, and then I stopped
- ❏ I honored my "I've had enough" signals
- ❏ I stayed off the scale

FAST CHECK-IN

Rate the difficulty of today's fast on a scale from 1 to 10 (circle one):

1   2   3   4   5   6   7   8   9   **10**

(Today was easy! I sailed right through it.)   (Today was HARD! I struggled.)

During today's fast, I felt _____

_____

_____

_____

_____

_____

(*examples: exhilarated, hopeful, hungry, uncomfortable, bored, etc.*)

I used these strategies to manage my feelings today (check all that apply and add your own):

- ❏ I remembered my *why*
- ❏ I stayed busy
- ❏ I enjoyed a clean-fast-safe beverage
- ❏ I went on a walk
- ❏ I imagined my body tapping into my fat stores for fuel
- ❏ _____
  _____
- ❏ _____
  _____
- ❏ _____
  _____

EATING WINDOW CHECK-IN

Eating Window Length Goal: _____ hours
Actual Eating Window Length: _____ hours

How do I feel about today's eating window?

_____
_____
_____
_____
_____
_____
_____
_____
_____

What went well? Was there anything that I struggled with during my eating window? _____

_____

_____

_____

_____

_____

_____

_____

_____

TODAY'S NSVS, OR NON-SCALE VICTORIES

One of the most powerful things we can do is acknowledge our Non-Scale Victories (NSVs). These can be physical (*pain reduction, better energy, mental clarity, etc.*) or emotional (*freedom around food, confidence, etc.*).

What were today's NSVs? _____

_____

_____

_____

_____

_____

_____

_____

REFLECTIONS

Today, I listened to my body when I: _____

_____

_____

_____

_____

_____

_____

Today's *AHA!* moment(s): _____

_____

_____

_____

Something that is on my mind: _____

_____

_____

_____

PREPARING FOR SUCCESS

Goal(s) and/or strategies for tomorrow: _____

_____

_____

_____

_____

_____

DAY 9: LET'S FLIP THAT METABOLIC SWITCH— *OPERATION GLYCOGEN DEPLETION*

Today's Date: _____

PLANNING FOR A SUCCESSFUL DAY 9

Today, I am following

❑ The *Easy Does It* Approach (ten-hour window, low-carb ease-in breakfast or early lunch, low-carb ease-in snack, plus a regular dinner)

❑ The *Steady Build* Approach (seven-hour window, including lunch and dinner)

❑ The *Rip Off the Band-Aid* Approach (six-hour window, including lunch *or* snack, and dinner)

My personal goal(s) for today: _____

_____

_____

_____

_____

Daily Lesson from Gin: Let's flip that metabolic switch— *Operation Glycogen Depletion.*

This is one of the more science-y sections of the book, and it's important. I'm going to teach you the basics of what's going on in your body during the adjustment period as you become fat adapted and why the physical adaptations feel like such a struggle at times. I promise it gets easier! (If it didn't, none of us could live an intermittent fasting lifestyle long term.)

Keep in mind that I'm simplifying what are very complex processes (and there are lots of other processes happening simultaneously), but understanding your "metabolic switch" can help you understand some of the challenges you'll face while your body is adapting to the clean fast, and you'll be confident that you can get through the tough parts to the smooth sailing that awaits you on the other side.

When fasting, we are able to ignite our bodies' fat-burning superpower by "flipping the metabolic switch," a term I first heard in a 2018 paper about fasting that was published in the journal *Obesity*. That term helped me immediately understand what was going on in our bodies in a new way: we need to flip that metabolic switch before fasting feels "easy." Keep reading to understand why and also understand when it happens.

When the metabolic switch is flipped, our bodies go from running on glucose (from the foods we eat and our stored glycogen) to running on the fat from our fat cells and also the ketones that are produced to fuel our brains. It may surprise you to learn that our bodies are able to get into ketosis during the fast, and it happens once we are fat adapted.

Yes, it's true. When the metabolic switch is flipped, we are able to produce ketones while fasting even if we are not following a ketogenic diet during our eating window! It all has to do with the level of glycogen stores in our liver.

At what point do our bodies flip this metabolic switch and become fat adapted? It happens when our liver glycogen has been sufficiently depleted and fat cells are mobilized to meet

9

our energy needs. It usually occurs at some point between hours twelve and thirty-six of fasting, and this completely depends on how much glycogen is stored in someone's liver as well as how much energy that person is using throughout the day (as an example, exercise uses energy and helps us flip the switch sooner).

Think of the liver as a glycogen storage tank (*the liver is a lot more than a glycogen tank, but visualizing it as a storage tank helps you understand what is happening*).

Let's say someone begins IF with full liver glycogen stores. The tank is full. That person won't use it all up (or get into ketosis) that day, or even necessarily for the first few weeks of their intermittent fasting lifestyle. However, every day, that person will deplete some of her glycogen stores during the fast. Every day, if she is fasting long enough, she depletes more than her body adds back during the eating window, even if she is eating carbs. (Not all your glucose goes into glycogen storage after you eat, by the way. Some of it is used for immediate energy needs.)

Over time, thanks to the clean fast, she takes out more glycogen each day than she puts back in, and through the daily fasting periods, the amount of stored liver glycogen gets lower and lower day by day. The level in the storage tank goes down slowly.

Eventually, after fasting clean for as many daily fasts as it takes her to deplete her glycogen stores sufficiently, glycogen stores are low enough that her body needs to find another fuel source for the brain. Her body switches over to fat burning, and ketosis kicks in. BOOM! The metabolic switch has been flipped! The brain is happy, because there is now a steady supply of ketones produced from stored fat.

Our brains *love* ketones, and once we have a steady supply, we experience amazing mental clarity and increased energy during the fast! This is one of my favorite features of living an intermittent fasting lifestyle.

Once your body learns to tap into your fat for fuel during the fast, you reach a state we call *metabolic flexibility*, and I believe it is how our bodies are meant to function. (In fact, metabolic *in*flexibility is linked to many of the diseases that are plaguing modern society, such as metabolic syndrome, type 2 diabetes, cancer, as well as other age-related diseases.)

What does metabolic flexibility look like in our bodies? When we eat, we use food for fuel. When we fast, we switch over to using our backup fuel sources for energy, including our stored fat. Voilà! Metabolic flexibility, just as nature intended! This would have been important in the past when we didn't have a grocery store or fast-food restaurant on every corner, or a pantry fully stocked with snacks. Our survival would have depended on our bodies' ability to switch fuel sources as needed. Regaining this flexibility is *huge*.

Here is what is REALLY important to understand: we don't regain this metabolic flexibility overnight. It takes time.

Think of how we have to build up our endurance when we begin a new exercise regimen, and that should help you understand what I mean. If you wanted to run a 5K, but you had been sedentary for years, you wouldn't be able to run the 5K on day 1. You might decide to complete a couch-to-5K program, where you would gradually build up your physical endurance from day to day, until one day, you can run a 5K without stopping.

9

Think of the IF adjustment period in a similar way. We have to "build up our fasting muscle" over time. Picture your liver glycogen gradually draining away, and know that you'll feel better soon.

You're reading this on day 9, and you may be wondering where you are in the process. Unfortunately, that varies from person to person. The 28-Day FAST Start is designed so that most new Ifers will flip that metabolic switch by day 28, but it can be sooner (or later) for some. If you have been metabolically unhealthy for a while, it will likely take you longer to adapt than a body that is already metabolically healthy.

As you continue to go along from day to day, you may find that fasting gets harder again before it gets easier. This is normal. It's actually a good sign when that happens, because it indicates your body is just about to flip the metabolic switch.

Suddenly, the storage tank is getting low. You're getting to the end of the glycogen stores that your body has been using for energy during the fast. Now, your body needs to switch over to fat burning for fuel.

You may feel like you're moving through Jell-O for a few days just before the switch is flipped. Hang in there! Once the transition happens, you'll feel better. Fasting becomes easier, and you'll have more energy.

In fact, when you find over the coming days or weeks that you're struggling, that's when to get excited, because you know you're about to ignite your fat-burning superpower!

DAILY INSPIRATION SPOTLIGHT:
Tish Times, Phoenix, Arizona
Intermittent Fasting Stories guest, episode 275

How long has she been an intermittent faster? *Between three and four years.*

I originally found intermittent fasting because I was diagnosed with diverticulitis. I had been out sick quite a bit, in and out of the hospital, and when I posted on Facebook about it, several people messaged me with stories about their own experiences. Some were providing encouragement, others horror stories, but one person told me that I should try fasting. I really wish I remembered her name, but just the mention of it was life-changing. I eventually started reading books and listening to podcasts. I heard a podcast featuring Kim Smith (episode 1 of Intermittent Fasting Stories*) and she referred to Gin's book* Delay, Don't Deny. *I purchased it right away. I joined the Facebook group and purchased anything Gin had written at the time. Although I had been fasting several months by the time I found the book, the book changed my life. Through* Delay, Don't Deny, *I learned about clean fasting and found a community. Because I learned about intermittent fasting, dozens of my friends and family began fasting, too. I have referred or shared* Delay, Don't Deny *or* Fast. Feast. Repeat. *so many times, and I continue to do so. Although I lost fifty-five pounds and had a tremendous life change due to intermittent fasting, I continued to battle against diverticulitis and eventually had to have a colon resection surgery. I firmly believe that I didn't need the surgery sooner because*

9

I had such a great health improvement through IF. After a successful surgery and recovery, I continued to use IF as part of my healing process. My doctors agreed that fasting played a part in my very quick recovery. I am continuing to fast consistently, and I am healthier than I've been in a decade. I've been able to maintain my weight loss and continue to move toward my ultimate goal. My life will never be the same since I've committed to a fasted lifestyle, and I am forever grateful for that person who messaged me on Facebook.

ADVICE FROM TISH

To anyone who is hesitant to start intermittent fasting or has stepped away from IF, I would say: There is no time like the present to change your life. You are only one decision away from changing your life. Make the decision now, then decide every day to put yourself and your health first. You can't control everything, but you can control when and how often you eat. Choose you . . . Do it now.

**YOU HAVE ALL THE TOOLS YOU NEED TO SUCCEED.
ENJOY YOUR DAY! YOU'VE GOT THIS.**

HOW DID IT GO?
IT'S TIME TO REFLECT ON DAY 9.

TODAY (CHECK ALL THAT APPLY):

❏ I fasted clean (plain water, unflavored sparkling water, black unflavored coffee, plain tea)
❏ During the fast, I took time to reflect on the positive changes happening in my body
❏ Within my eating window, I ate until I was satisfied, and then I stopped
❏ I honored my "I've had enough" signals
❏ I stayed off the scale

FAST CHECK-IN

Rate the difficulty of today's fast on a scale from 1 to 10 (circle one):

1 2 3 4 5 6 7 8 9 **10**

(Today was easy! I sailed right through it.)   (Today was HARD! I struggled.)

During today's fast, I felt _____

_____

_____

_____

_____

_____

(*examples: exhilarated, hopeful, hungry, uncomfortable, bored, etc.*)

I used these strategies to manage my feelings today (check all that apply and add your own):

- ❏ I remembered my *why*
- ❏ I stayed busy
- ❏ I enjoyed a clean-fast-safe beverage
- ❏ I went on a walk
- ❏ I imagined my body tapping into my fat stores for fuel
- ❏ _____
  _____
- ❏ _____
  _____
- ❏ _____
  _____

EATING WINDOW CHECK-IN

Eating Window Length Goal: _____ hours
Actual Eating Window Length: _____ hours

How do I feel about today's eating window?

_____
_____
_____
_____
_____
_____
_____
_____
_____

What went well? Was there anything that I struggled with during my eating window? _____

_____
_____
_____
_____
_____
_____
_____
_____
_____

TODAY'S NSVS, OR NON-SCALE VICTORIES

One of the most powerful things we can do is acknowledge our Non-Scale Victories (NSVs). These can be physical (*pain reduction, better energy, mental clarity, etc.*) or emotional (*freedom around food, confidence, etc.*).

What were today's NSVs? _____

_____
_____
_____
_____
_____
_____
_____
_____

REFLECTIONS

Today, I listened to my body when I: _____

_____

_____

_____

_____

_____

_____

_____

Today's *AHA!* moment(s): _____

_____

_____

_____

Something that is on my mind: _____

_____

_____

_____

PREPARING FOR SUCCESS

Goal(s) and/or strategies for tomorrow: _____

_____

_____

_____

_____

DAY 10: HELP! I CAN'T SLEEP!

Today's Date: _____

PLANNING FOR A SUCCESSFUL DAY 10

Today, I am following

- ❏ The *Easy Does It* Approach (ten-hour window, low-carb ease-in breakfast or early lunch, low-carb ease-in snack, plus a regular dinner)
- ❏ The *Steady Build* Approach (seven-hour window, including lunch and dinner)
- ❏ The *Rip Off the Band-Aid* Approach (six-hour window, including lunch *or* snack, and dinner)

My personal goal(s) for today: _____

_____

_____

_____

_____

Daily Lesson from Gin: Help! I can't sleep!

I do hear this from time to time, especially from new IFers. The good news is that this phase generally passes quickly after your body adapts to fasting.

So why does it happen? Think back to what you learned yesterday.

10

After your body becomes fat adapted, you begin producing ketones for fuel. This is a powerful source of energy, especially for your brain.

The downside is that you may suddenly feel wired and unable to settle down, especially at night.

After your body adjusts to this new fuel source, the sensation of feeling wired won't be as pronounced. You'll notice increased mental clarity during the day (versus your pre-IF life), but you'll finally be able to sleep again.

Even after you become adapted, however, you may find that certain things negatively affect your sleep.

Over time, experiment with different daily eating windows and foods to see what works best for you. As an example, I sleep better when I eat sufficient starchy carbs and have an evening eating window, but I do not sleep well if I have too much sugar or too much wine. I also find that if I don't eat enough during my daily eating window, I don't sleep as well.

You may be the opposite: you may find that you sleep better when your eating window closes a few hours before bed, and maybe you need to eat fewer carbs to sleep well.

Throughout this entire process, never forget that you are a study of one. Tune in to your body, and know that you have the power to figure out what works best for you. My ideal eating window may not be the same as your ideal eating window.

One other thing I do that helps my body relax at night is to take a high-quality magnesium supplement at bedtime. I don't take many supplements, because I prefer to meet my nutritional needs through foods when I can, but much of our soil is depleted of magnesium in today's modern world, and many of us are magnesium deficient as a result of this. Consider adding a magnesium supplement and see if that helps.

DAILY INSPIRATION SPOTLIGHT:
Paul Hunter, Nashville, Tennessee
Intermittent Fasting Stories guest, episode 54

How long has he been an intermittent faster? *Between four and five years.*

When I was on the podcast, I had been fasting for a little over a year and a half, and I had reached my goal weight. I had lost a total of 54 pounds with intermittent fasting using 16:8 for a year and then switching to a 21:3, because it just felt better at that point. Since the episode aired in November of 2019, a lot has changed. We went through the pandemic. Both of my daughters got married. I now have a grandson. I made a couple of job changes, and then I went back to the company I've worked for now for seventeen years. Through all those changes, one thing hasn't changed: my intermittent fasting. I still fast every single day. Most days, I have a three-hour eating window. Some days it's two hours, some days it's five or six, but usually right around three. I still maintain my goal weight. I like to stay within a few pounds of 177 pounds, and for the first time in my life, I've done it now for several years in a row. I still train in jujitsu four or five days a week. I keep up with guys that are twenty or thirty years younger than I am. I have so many friends who I've inspired to start fasting that have stuck with it, and that gives me great joy. I know how it changed my life, and I love watching it change other people's lives as well. I will never go back to eating multiple meals per day.

10

ADVICE FROM PAUL

I would say, "Trust the process, and don't quit." You will go through ups and downs. You'll have stretches that are difficult, but if you stick to the process, you'll get through those and get back to those times when it feels great.

**YOU HAVE ALL THE TOOLS YOU NEED TO SUCCEED.
ENJOY YOUR DAY! YOU'VE GOT THIS.**

HOW DID IT GO?
IT'S TIME TO REFLECT ON DAY 10.

TODAY (CHECK ALL THAT APPLY):

❏ I fasted clean (plain water, unflavored sparkling water, black unflavored coffee, plain tea)
❏ During the fast, I took time to reflect on the positive changes happening in my body
❏ Within my eating window, I ate until I was satisfied, and then I stopped
❏ I honored my "I've had enough" signals
❏ I stayed off the scale

FAST CHECK-IN

Rate the difficulty of today's fast on a scale from 1 to 10 (circle one):

1   2   3   4   5   6   7   8   9   **10**

(Today was easy! I sailed right through it.)   (Today was HARD! I struggled.)

During today's fast, I felt _____
_____
_____
_____
_____
_____

(*examples: exhilarated, hopeful, hungry, uncomfortable, bored, etc.*)

I used these strategies to manage my feelings today (check all that apply and add your own):

- ❑ I remembered my *why*
- ❑ I stayed busy
- ❑ I enjoyed a clean-fast-safe beverage
- ❑ I went on a walk
- ❑ I imagined my body tapping into my fat stores for fuel
- ❑ _____
  _____
- ❑ _____
  _____
- ❑ _____
  _____

EATING WINDOW CHECK-IN

Eating Window Length Goal: _____ hours
Actual Eating Window Length: _____ hours

How do I feel about today's eating window?

_____
_____
_____
_____
_____
_____
_____
_____
_____
_____

What went well? Was there anything that I struggled with during my eating window? _____

_____

_____

_____

_____

_____

_____

_____

_____

_____

TODAY'S NSVS, OR NON-SCALE VICTORIES

One of the most powerful things we can do is acknowledge our Non-Scale Victories (NSVs). These can be physical (*pain reduction, better energy, mental clarity, etc.*) or emotional (*freedom around food, confidence, etc.*).

What were today's NSVs? _____

_____

_____

_____

_____

_____

_____

_____

_____

REFLECTIONS

Today, I listened to my body when I: _____

_____

_____

_____

_____

_____

_____

_____

Today's *AHA!* moment(s): _____

_____

_____

_____

Something that is on my mind: _____

_____

_____

_____

PREPARING FOR SUCCESS

Goal(s) and/or strategies for tomorrow: _____

_____

_____

_____

_____

DAY 11: HELP! I'M OVEREATING. THIS ISN'T GOING TO WORK. . . .

Today's Date: _____

PLANNING FOR A SUCCESSFUL DAY 11

Today, I am following

❏ The *Easy Does It* Approach (ten-hour window, low-carb ease-in breakfast or early lunch, low-carb ease-in snack, plus a regular dinner)
❏ The *Steady Build* Approach (seven-hour window, including lunch and dinner)
❏ The *Rip Off the Band-Aid* Approach (six-hour window, including lunch *or* snack, and dinner)

My personal goal(s) for today: _____

_____

_____

_____

_____

Daily Lesson from Gin: Help! I'm overeating. This isn't going to work. . . .

Today's lesson is really important, because many new IFers become panicked when they begin IF and find that when their window opens, it feels like the floodgates have opened. How in the world is IF going to be a successful weight-loss strategy if you are bingeing every time your window opens?

11

During the FAST Start, never forget that your body is learning how to do something new. Before you started IF, you were likely someone who ate frequently during the day . . . After all, that is what we have been told to do. We have all heard the advice to eat frequent small meals throughout the day to lose weight. (Why in the world did we think that eating *more frequently* would be a successful weight-loss strategy?)

The result is that your body became used to frequent fuelings during the day. Running low on easily accessible fuel? Your body sends you the message: "Time to eat!" And you send some more fuel down in the form of a snack or a meal. Never mind that there is plenty of fuel stored on your body for later in the form of excess body fat. Your body doesn't want to do the work it takes to tap into that stored fuel when you can simply send more easily accessible fuel down at any given moment.

But now, you've started fasting . . . and your body is confused.

Remember what you learned on day 9: first, your body uses up your stored glycogen, and then it needs to find another source of fuel. It takes time for your body to become fat adapted, and before that metabolic switch is flipped, you're not accessing your fat stores efficiently. So, your body is HUNGRY.

As a result, you get the signal to eat and eat when your window opens. This is why many people don't lose weight during the adjustment period or may even gain weight.

But! Once your body adjusts to the fast in a few weeks, your body will have access to plenty of fuel during the fast . . . your stored body fat! And the urge to overeat goes away.

The takeaway: if you feel like you are overdoing it in your eating window, know that it is normal to be extra-hungry while your body adjusts to fasting. Hang in there, and do NOT beat yourself up over it. This stage will pass.

DAILY INSPIRATION SPOTLIGHT:
Laurie Lewis, Portland, Oregon
Intermittent Fasting Stories guest, episode 4 and episode 115

How long has she been an intermittent faster? *Over five years.*

Wailing like a five-year-old, I let my mother know she was wrong! I was doing everything I could to address the menopausal fifty-plus pounds I had gained. I'd reached rock bottom and had just about given up hope. I was aching head to toe, and my mind was foggy and forgetful. I felt despondent and furious that I couldn't find a solution, and she quietly listened and offered to pray for an answer. That night, I researched (yet again!) "stubborn, hormonal, menopause fat, lose weight now help me," and up popped a term I'd never heard before. Intermittent fasting. What surprised me was I'd been studying nutrition and health for over twenty years, so why was this unfamiliar? I stayed up late to learn more, and the next morning, I gleefully shared that maybe I'd found an answer. When I explained it to her, Mom responded that it made perfect sense and asked how she could support me. Thank goodness I like black coffee, and I started that very same day. Some days, it took some effort, and all days, it made me feel confident and proud that I could take control of my health and put my body into a fat-burning state of repair. My eating windows varied, and after a few months, I settled into a 20:4 schedule. This regimen made me feel so well, and the body pain subsided, brain fog cleared, plantar

11

fasciitis went away, and I had great energy all day for my athletic pursuits and work. Pretty quickly, people around me started noticing my happier spirit and healthier body. Everyone wanted to know how, and when a group of friends cornered me at a wedding, I agreed to put together an online class. I would not wait until January, though; we would begin now! It was important I show them that people can have an eating window under any circumstances, at any time. There's no reason to treat November and December as a free-for-all and then use January to fix it. Right from the beginning of my Fast Forward Wellness coaching business, I led people away from the prison of diet culture and diet mindset, into the freedom of curiosity, discovery, choice, and celebration. Guiding women through the chaos of perimenopause, the confusion of menopause, and the worries of health and aging has been the astonishing outcome of deciding one day to have an eating window. Imagine how full my heart is that after all my struggle, I get to show women around the world their very bright futures with intermittent fasting as the foundation!

ADVICE FROM LAURIE

You cannot mess this up. Lean in with curiosity and make the choice to develop a communion WITH your body. Decide that your daily fasting hours are your "healing hours," and then fully enjoy delicious food later in your eating window. This isn't something to stop and start; every day, you have an eating window— and YOU get to say when it is!

YOU HAVE ALL THE TOOLS YOU NEED TO SUCCEED. ENJOY YOUR DAY! YOU'VE GOT THIS.

HOW DID IT GO?
IT'S TIME TO REFLECT ON DAY 11.

TODAY (CHECK ALL THAT APPLY):

❏ I fasted clean (plain water, unflavored sparkling water, black unflavored coffee, plain tea)
❏ During the fast, I took time to reflect on the positive changes happening in my body
❏ Within my eating window, I ate until I was satisfied, and then I stopped
❏ I honored my "I've had enough" signals
❏ I stayed off the scale

FAST CHECK-IN

Rate the difficulty of today's fast on a scale from 1 to 10 (circle one):

1　2　3　4　5　6　7　8　9　**10**

(Today was easy! I sailed right through it.)　　(Today was HARD! I struggled.)

During today's fast, I felt _____
_____
_____
_____
_____
_____

(*examples: exhilarated, hopeful, hungry, uncomfortable, bored, etc.*)

I used these strategies to manage my feelings today (check all that apply and add your own):

- ❏ I remembered my *why*
- ❏ I stayed busy
- ❏ I enjoyed a clean-fast-safe beverage
- ❏ I went on a walk
- ❏ I imagined my body tapping into my fat stores for fuel
- ❏ _____
  _____
- ❏ _____
  _____
- ❏ _____
  _____

EATING WINDOW CHECK-IN

Eating Window Length Goal: _____ hours
Actual Eating Window Length: _____ hours

How do I feel about today's eating window?

_____
_____
_____
_____
_____
_____
_____
_____
_____

What went well? Was there anything that I struggled with during my eating window? _____

_____

_____

_____

_____

_____

_____

_____

_____

_____

_____

TODAY'S NSVS, OR NON-SCALE VICTORIES

One of the most powerful things we can do is acknowledge our Non-Scale Victories (NSVs). These can be physical (*pain reduction, better energy, mental clarity, etc.*) or emotional (*freedom around food, confidence, etc.*).

What were today's NSVs? _____

_____

_____

_____

_____

_____

_____

_____

_____

REFLECTIONS

Today, I listened to my body when I: _____

_____

_____

_____

_____

_____

_____

_____

Today's *AHA!* moment(s): _____

_____

_____

_____

_____

Something that is on my mind: _____

_____

_____

_____

_____

PREPARING FOR SUCCESS

Goal(s) and/or strategies for tomorrow: _____

_____

_____

_____

_____

DAY 12: LIFESTYLE VERSUS DIET— WHAT'S THE DIFFERENCE?

Today's Date: _____

PLANNING FOR A SUCCESSFUL DAY 12

Today, I am following

❏ The *Easy Does It* Approach (ten-hour window, low-carb ease-in breakfast or early lunch, low-carb ease-in snack, plus a regular dinner)
❏ The *Steady Build* Approach (seven-hour window, including lunch and dinner)
❏ The *Rip Off the Band-Aid* Approach (six-hour window, including lunch *or* snack, and dinner)

My personal goal(s) for today: _____

_____

_____

_____

_____

Daily Lesson from Gin: Lifestyle versus diet—what's the difference?

You'll never hear me talk about the "intermittent fasting diet." IF is *not* a diet!

I bet every time you read a diet book, they told you, "*This isn't a diet! It's a lifestyle!*" And yet, when you began

12

reading the plan, it became clear that you were going on a diet.

And here I am, telling you the same thing about intermittent fasting.

So how do you know the difference? What's the difference between a diet and a lifestyle?

Your "diet" is what you eat. We all have "a diet," even if you don't realize it or name it. Maybe you're someone who eats the Standard American Diet (most people in the U.S. eat that way). Or maybe you eat according to other guidelines that you enjoy following.

When you *go on* "a diet," which most of us have done at some point in the past, it is focused on changing the *what*. Maybe you were eating the Standard American Diet and realized that it wasn't working for you, so you decided to try something else to see if it worked better for you. (Spoiler alert: most eating styles work better than the Standard American Diet, also known as the SAD, which says it all . . .)

Here are just a few examples of diets you may have heard of or tried:

- Keto diet: You follow a ketogenic eating plan.
- Vegan diet: You eat only foods that are free of animal products.
- Paleo diet: You choose foods that (theoretically) were available in Paleolithic times.
- Whole 30 diet: You eliminate certain foods deemed to be potentially problematic and focus only on whole foods for thirty days.
- Mediterranean diet: You focus on foods that are common in the Mediterranean region.

When you think about that list, you see that diet plans are centered around what you can or should eat, and most diets also include lists or categories of foods that you should avoid.

Intermittent fasting, on the other hand, is not about *what*. It's about *when*.

We structure our intermittent fasting lifestyle around periods of time when we are fasting and periods of time when we are eating.

When you live an intermittent fasting lifestyle, you get to decide what you eat in your eating window. Whether you follow the Standard American Diet or any other eating style is totally up to you.

As I told you on day 6, you get to eat whatever *you* want.

During your FAST Start, it's best not to make too many changes at once. This means that it's usually best to make no changes to your diet as you begin living an IF lifestyle. When we change both the *when* and the *what* at the same time, it can lead to burnout and you're more likely to quit in frustration. Remember, we are here to make sure your IF lifestyle *sticks*.

When I began living an IF lifestyle in 2014, I definitely followed the Standard American Diet. Now, the foods I crave are entirely different. It happened naturally, and I didn't have to force it.

You'll get better at listening to your body as time goes on, and this generally changes the foods we want to eat. It's almost universally true that most of us gravitate to a different "diet" over time than we came in with.

Am I telling you that you will eventually need to "go on a diet" while you're an IFer? Absolutely not.

But be prepared to be delighted with how your tastes

12

change over the coming months and years. (It won't happen by tomorrow . . . so be patient, and pay attention.)

DAILY INSPIRATION SPOTLIGHT:
Graeme Currie, Perth, Western Australia
Intermittent Fasting Stories guest, episode 23 and episode 206

How long has he been an intermittent faster? *Between four and five years.*

Gin's podcast was my coming-out in terms of talking about my past issues with sugar and fast-food addiction. The reaction to my story was overwhelming and a big surprise to me; I got messages from people all over the world who resonated with my story. Since that podcast, I went on to author a book, The Fasting Highway, *an Amazon category bestseller and multi-category number one new release. I started my own podcast of the same name. My desire to share my passion for intermittent fasting also led me to create my online Facebook community, also called the Fasting Highway and Book. Some eight thousand people from around the world quickly joined the community. Since I was on Gin's podcast, I have been a guest on other podcasts sharing my story and experiences with intermittent fasting. After losing 60 kilograms (132 pounds) over fifteen months, I have successfully maintained that weight loss coming up on four years. Gin's podcast lit the fire within me to share my story to the world. I have built up an amazing band of followers in every corner of the world since I was on the podcast back in 2019. I now consider Gin a friend, and I am eternally grateful for the chance to share my story on the* Intermittent Fasting Stories *podcast.*

ADVICE FROM GRAEME

Start slowly and stay in your comfort zone. Do not compare to others, as you are the experiment of one. Stay plugged into a good online community, and read everything that Gin Stephens and Dr. Jason Fung put out. Nail the clean fast, and eat what makes you feel your greatest, not what your mind wants. Listen to as many podcasts on IF as you can.

**YOU HAVE ALL THE TOOLS YOU NEED TO SUCCEED.
ENJOY YOUR DAY! YOU'VE GOT THIS.**

12

HOW DID IT GO?
IT'S TIME TO REFLECT ON DAY 12.

TODAY (CHECK ALL THAT APPLY):

- ❏ I fasted clean (plain water, unflavored sparkling water, black unflavored coffee, plain tea)
- ❏ During the fast, I took time to reflect on the positive changes happening in my body
- ❏ Within my eating window, I ate until I was satisfied, and then I stopped
- ❏ I honored my "I've had enough" signals
- ❏ I stayed off the scale

FAST CHECK-IN

Rate the difficulty of today's fast on a scale from 1 to 10 (circle one):

1 2 3 4 5 6 7 8 9 **10**

(Today was easy! I sailed right through it.)   (Today was HARD! I struggled.)

During today's fast, I felt _____

_____

_____

_____

_____

_____

(*examples: exhilarated, hopeful, hungry, uncomfortable, bored, etc.*)

I used these strategies to manage my feelings today (check all that apply and add your own):

❏ I remembered my *why*
❏ I stayed busy
❏ I enjoyed a clean-fast-safe beverage
❏ I went on a walk
❏ I imagined my body tapping into my fat stores for fuel
❏ _____

❏ _____

❏ _____

EATING WINDOW CHECK-IN

Eating Window Length Goal: _____ hours
Actual Eating Window Length: _____ hours

How do I feel about today's eating window?

_____
_____
_____
_____
_____
_____
_____
_____
_____

What went well? Was there anything that I struggled with during my eating window? _____

_____

_____

_____

_____

_____

_____

_____

_____

_____

TODAY'S NSVS, OR NON-SCALE VICTORIES

One of the most powerful things we can do is acknowledge our Non-Scale Victories (NSVs). These can be physical (*pain reduction, better energy, mental clarity, etc.*) or emotional (*freedom around food, confidence, etc.*).

What were today's NSVs? _____

_____

_____

_____

_____

_____

_____

_____

_____

REFLECTIONS

Today, I listened to my body when I: _____

_____

_____

_____

_____

_____

_____

_____

_____

Today's *AHA!* moment(s): _____

_____

_____

_____

_____

Something that is on my mind: _____

_____

_____

_____

_____

PREPARING FOR SUCCESS

Goal(s) and/or strategies for tomorrow: _____

_____

_____

_____

_____

_____

DAY 13: YOU *CAN* DO HARD THINGS!

Today's Date: _____

PLANNING FOR A SUCCESSFUL DAY 13

Today, I am following

❑ The *Easy Does It* Approach (ten-hour window, low-carb ease-in breakfast or early lunch, low-carb ease-in snack, plus a regular dinner)

❑ The *Steady Build* Approach (seven-hour window, including lunch and dinner)

❑ The *Rip Off the Band-Aid* Approach (six-hour window, including lunch *or* snack, and dinner)

My personal goal(s) for today: _____

_____

_____

_____

_____

_____

Daily Lesson from Gin: You CAN do hard things!

As you progress through the adjustment period of the FAST Start, you may find that the newness starts to wear off. You were SO EXCITED on day 1 (or even in week 1), and the sheer excitement of living a new lifestyle kept you going.

Day by day, however, resentment may set in.

I get it. I've been there!

- Maybe your family is eating breakfast while you're fasting . . . and even worse, it's food YOU had to prepare for them.

- Or maybe your skinny friend at the office is having another chicken biscuit in front of you. Or everyone is eating doughnuts at a meeting. And YOU "have to" sit there and fast.

- Perhaps you're at the coffee shop and the person in front of you orders your favorite seasonal latte, and all YOU get is boring black coffee.

"Why is this so HARD, Gin???"

It's "hard" because we are used to eating for so many more reasons than hunger. Food is everywhere. It keeps us company when we are lonely. It entertains us when we are bored. It connects us when we share a meal with friends or loved ones.

When you have the feelings that "this is hard," sit with those feelings and *feel them.*

There is a saying I'm sure you have heard before:

Dieting is hard. Being overweight is hard. Pick your hard.

I just got through telling you on day 12 that intermittent fasting isn't a diet, and I meant it. But that familiar saying can apply to IF, as well, with just a few wording changes:

Fasting (rather than finding comfort through eating) will sometimes be hard. Living the way you used to live was hard. Pick your hard.

Here's the truth: living an intermittent fasting lifestyle isn't easy every moment of every day. I'm not going to tell you that it is.

BUT! It is *so much easier than how we used to live.*

13

When intermittent fasting feels hard—and sometimes it will—remind yourself of the alternatives:

- You could go on another restrictive diet where you have to count calories or points or grams of things.
- You could take the NEW! "miracle" weight-loss shot/drug/supplement your friend is raving about . . . along with all the expense and side effects that come along with it, plus the weight gain that always happens when you stop taking it.
- You could simply give up and decide that you're destined to be overweight and miserable.
- You could have weight-loss surgery and permanently alter your body and your digestion.

Not a single one of those options is *easy*.

In comparison to that list of options, I think we would all agree that intermittent fasting is *much easier*.

All you have to do is *delay*.

- When you're craving that creamy cup of coffee, *delay it*. You can have it later.
- When there are doughnuts in the break room, grab one for later and *delay it*. You can still have that doughnut . . . if you even want it by the time your window opens (most of the time, you won't).
- When your friend wants to go out for breakfast, ask if you can meet for a late lunch instead: *delay it*!

Once you master the delay, even the hard moments won't feel as hard.

The answer isn't *no* . . . it's *not yet*.

And never forget:
*You **can** do hard things.*

DAILY INSPIRATION SPOTLIGHT:
Jamie, Hinesburg, Vermont
Intermittent Fasting Stories guest, episode 219

How long has she been an intermittent faster? *Between two and three years.*

My weight has been a challenge for me since childhood. I was born in the late 1970s, when processed foods were the norm and food pyramid the guide to a healthy diet. I spent a majority of my life dieting and exercising to maintain my weight. I tried Nutrisystem, WeightWatchers, South Beach, and Beach Body, to name a few, and spent too much money in the process. In 2018, at a routine appointment, the nurse practitioner noted I had an enlarged thyroid. Upon further testing by my primary doctor, it was discovered I had a "normal" TSH (3.8), but extremely high TPO antibodies (>1,300) leading to diagnosis of Hashimoto's (an autoimmune thyroid disease). I had symptoms of hypothyroidism but attributed them to being a tired mom of three little kids. What mom isn't tired with headaches? It was the bone-chilling cold and brain fog I described and the elevated TPO antibodies that prompted my doctor to try levothyroxine, a once-daily medication, for my hypothyroidism. I thought maybe this would be the "magic pill" and answer to my weight struggles. Well, it wasn't, and I

13

continued to battle my weight and knew I could feel better. Although I considered myself a "healthy eater," I connected with a nutritionist in hopes she could offer me ideas to help me have more energy and maintain a healthy weight. It was then that I was first introduced to intermittent fasting. She didn't give me a ton of information, but basically encouraged me to eat in an eight-hour eating window. I did it and was able to maintain my weight, but felt it was too restrictive for my needs at the time, and drifted away from intermittent fasting after about six months. Enter the year 2020 and the pandemic. I was working as a nurse in health care, and my husband is a pharmacist, so while the world closed down, we continued working and trying to balance the needs of three kids at home with remote school and so many unknowns in the world. Without changing my diet, I gained about 10 pounds. In a chance encounter in the staff lounge at work, a moment I now call serendipity, I heard some coworkers talking about eating, weight loss, et cetera. I didn't have time to hear more, but my coworker Tiffani knew I was interested! Thankfully, she reached out to me via a Facebook message: "Jamie—don't buy anything for weight loss! Read the book Delay, Don't Deny *by Gin Stephens and then* The Obesity Code *by Dr. Jason Fung. Those two books changed my life. Happy to help if you have any questions. I've been doing it for a year and a half. You won't regret it!" I had no expectations, only hopes to get the scale going in a better direction, so I read* Delay, Don't Deny. *It ALL grabbed me and made so much sense this time. I hit the ground running, quickly learned how to listen to my body in the quietness of the fast, and found so much freedom in intermittent fasting. In ten months, I lost 50 pounds, I felt more energetic, and I knew I had found a* lifestyle that was meant for me. I made IF into something flexible—what I needed for my life on any given day, not what someone else needed. Now, nearly three years later, I easily maintain my weight and never plan to sway from fasting. It has brought me more than weight loss; it has provided my body with peace, a true gift to myself. I'm five foot nine, and I started at 215 pounds. It took me ten months to lose 50 pounds, and now I easily maintain my weight around 160–165 pounds.

ADVICE FROM JAMIE

Think of intermittent fasting as a flexible lifestyle, not a short-term solution, and the rest will fall into place. Let your body be your guide, initially taking it one fast at a time. Set small goals for yourself over time, be it the length of your fast or a change in what you are eating. Listen to your body—it has incredible things to tell you in the quietness of the fast. We are all unique, and IF can be tweaked to make it a just-right fit for you. Give fasting a chance. Find your fasting tribe to support and cheer you on, and discover the freedom fasting provides . . . It's waiting for you.

YOU HAVE ALL THE TOOLS YOU NEED TO SUCCEED. ENJOY YOUR DAY! YOU'VE GOT THIS.

13

HOW DID IT GO?
IT'S TIME TO REFLECT ON DAY 13.

TODAY (CHECK ALL THAT APPLY):

❏ I fasted clean (plain water, unflavored sparkling water, black unflavored coffee, plain tea)
❏ During the fast, I took time to reflect on the positive changes happening in my body
❏ Within my eating window, I ate until I was satisfied, and then I stopped
❏ I honored my "I've had enough" signals
❏ I stayed off the scale

FAST CHECK-IN

Rate the difficulty of today's fast on a scale from 1 to 10 (circle one):

1　2　3　4　5　6　7　8　9　**10**

(Today was easy! I sailed right through it.)　　(Today was HARD! I struggled.)

During today's fast, I felt _____
_____
_____
_____
_____
_____

(*examples: exhilarated, hopeful, hungry, uncomfortable, bored, etc.*)

I used these strategies to manage my feelings today (check all that apply and add your own):

- ❏ I remembered my *why*
- ❏ I stayed busy
- ❏ I enjoyed a clean-fast-safe beverage
- ❏ I went on a walk
- ❏ I imagined my body tapping into my fat stores for fuel
- ❏ _____
  _____
- ❏ _____
  _____
- ❏ _____
  _____

EATING WINDOW CHECK-IN

Eating Window Length Goal: _____ hours
Actual Eating Window Length: _____ hours

How do I feel about today's eating window?

_____
_____
_____
_____
_____
_____
_____
_____
_____

What went well? Was there anything that I struggled with during my eating window? _____

_____

_____

_____

_____

_____

_____

_____

_____

_____

TODAY'S NSVS, OR NON-SCALE VICTORIES

One of the most powerful things we can do is acknowledge our Non-Scale Victories (NSVs). These can be physical (*pain reduction, better energy, mental clarity, etc.*) or emotional (*freedom around food, confidence, etc.*).

What were today's NSVs? _____

_____

_____

_____

_____

_____

_____

_____

REFLECTIONS

Today, I listened to my body when I: _____

_____

_____

_____

_____

_____

_____

_____

Today's *AHA!* moment(s): _____

_____

_____

_____

_____

Something that is on my mind: _____

_____

_____

_____

_____

PREPARING FOR SUCCESS

Goal(s) and/or strategies for tomorrow: _____

_____

_____

_____

_____

_____

DAY 14: WHAT DO I DO WITH ALL THIS EXTRA TIME?

Today's Date: _____

PLANNING FOR A SUCCESSFUL DAY 14

Today, I am following

- ❏ The *Easy Does It* Approach (ten-hour window, low-carb ease-in breakfast or early lunch, low-carb ease-in snack, plus a regular dinner)
- ❏ The *Steady Build* Approach (seven-hour window, including lunch and dinner)
- ❏ The *Rip Off the Band-Aid* Approach (six-hour window, including lunch *or* snack, and dinner)

My personal goal(s) for today: _____

_____

_____

_____

_____

_____

Daily Lesson from Gin: What do I do with all this extra time?

For some people, one of the most challenging parts of living an intermittent fasting lifestyle is that they don't know what to do with themselves.

We are so used to being food focused from the moment we wake up each day: breakfast, coffee breaks, snacks, lunch, more snacks, dinner, after-dinner snacks . . . the eating (and drinking) opportunities never seem to end.

As a new IFer, you may be missing the daily rituals that you'd become accustomed to. Pouring a mug of black coffee feels so stark in comparison to the joy you felt when adding all the ingredients you used to create your much-loved hot milkshake. And that hot milkshake felt like a hug in a mug, versus your boring and not-yet-delicious hot coffee-bean water.

And what do you do at mealtimes? If you work in an office, you are likely used to spending certain mealtimes with coworkers. If you're at home (with "frequent eaters" like your kids or your partner/spouse), they are eating multiple times per day while you are fasting.

Even if you're home alone, having snacks and meals gave you something to do and provided structure to your day.

Suddenly, the structure is gone, and you have to figure out something else to do.

When you are struggling with how to fill your typical snack time, coffee break time, or mealtime, there are lots of things you might choose to do instead, whether you are at home or at work. Here are just a few:

- Take a walk or have some other kind of movement break. (I have a rebounder that I love to jump on for a few minutes.)
- Run an errand.
- Talk to a friend.
- Turn on a podcast or some music and complete a task you've been putting off.
- Read a book. Maybe a chapter of *Fast. Feast. Repeat.*
- Heck, come to *this* book and read your daily lesson, or go back to a lesson you want to revisit.

14

It's all about developing new routines and habits. The longer you live an IF lifestyle, the easier it will become. It might be hard to believe, but trust me on this one.

One day, you'll look back and remember how much time you used to "waste" throughout your day worrying about the next snack or meal, and you'll realize how much more time IF gives you in your day. It's really a huge positive when you get to that point.

You'll get there!

DAILY INSPIRATION SPOTLIGHT:
Stephanie Gish, St. Petersburg, Florida
Intermittent Fasting Stories guest, episode 58

How long has she been an intermittent faster? *Between four and five years.*

In 2018, I gave fasting a second try after a failed attempt years before. I previously thought that I could just jump right in and start with a twenty-four-hour fast, but all I did was set myself up for failure. I didn't make it anywhere close to that. So, when I gave fasting another try in 2018, I started slowly by cutting out snacks, then skipped a meal, and eventually worked my way into a 16:8 intermittent fasting schedule. I started fasting as a way to help control my Crohn's disease symptoms and fight inflammation in my body. Now, I believe it is the most powerful tool in my arsenal for helping to heal my gut and improve my overall health and quality of life. As listeners of the Intermittent Fasting Stories *podcast may recall, it took me a year of fasting to finally realize I needed to do a clean fast. In 2019, I cut out the cream and sweeteners I was putting into my coffee and also worked my way up to longer fasting windows. By December of that year, I settled into an alternate-day fasting schedule. [Note from Gin: To learn more about the ADF approach, read the ADF chapter of* Fast. Feast. Repeat.*] At that time, my body needed the longer fasting periods to heal. Since then, however, I've been able to return to a 16:8 intermittent fasting protocol. I listened to my body over the years, and when it was ready for a shorter fasting window, I made the change. Fasting has continued to improve my relationship with food and overall gut health. I no longer worry about my diet and whether it will trigger Crohn's symptoms. My weight has remained the same, and I eat whatever I want; nothing is off-limits anymore. My diet is now filled with a variety of vegetables, meats, breads, and grains; I can even enjoy chocolate again! I try to limit sugar overall, but when I want dessert, I don't deny myself; I just make sure it's within my eating window. Since my episode aired in December 2019, I've also been able to manage my Crohn's disease well and have only experienced a few minor flare-ups that were most likely brought on by stress. Over the past few years, fasting has continued to get easier. I don't think about intermittent fasting as something I'm doing; it's just a part of how I live my life. Although it felt impossible the very first time I tried it, these days I usually forget that I'm actually fasting. I am grateful that I found my way back to intermittent fasting and for the opportunity to share my story.*

14

ADVICE FROM STEPHANIE

If you're ready to start fasting (or restart like I did), don't feel like you have to jump into the deep end. Start slowly by cutting out the snacks, and then skip a meal when you're ready. Let your body guide you. Intermittent fasting is a lifestyle for all the years ahead; you don't need to conquer it in a day. Keep searching for what works for you, and don't be afraid to shift your eating window earlier or later if that works better for you. Have patience and you'll find your personal fasting rhythm.

**YOU HAVE ALL THE TOOLS YOU NEED TO SUCCEED.
ENJOY YOUR DAY! YOU'VE GOT THIS.**

HOW DID IT GO?
IT'S TIME TO REFLECT ON DAY 14.

TODAY (CHECK ALL THAT APPLY):

- ❏ I fasted clean (plain water, unflavored sparkling water, black unflavored coffee, plain tea)
- ❏ During the fast, I took time to reflect on the positive changes happening in my body
- ❏ Within my eating window, I ate until I was satisfied, and then I stopped
- ❏ I honored my "I've had enough" signals
- ❏ I stayed off the scale

FAST CHECK-IN

Rate the difficulty of today's fast on a scale from 1 to 10 (circle one):

1   2   3   4   5   6   7   8   9   **10**

(Today was easy! I sailed right through it.)   (Today was HARD! I struggled.)

During today's fast, I felt _____
_____
_____
_____
_____
_____

(*examples: exhilarated, hopeful, hungry, uncomfortable, bored, etc.*)

I used these strategies to manage my feelings today (check all that apply and add your own):

- ❏ I remembered my *why*
- ❏ I stayed busy
- ❏ I enjoyed a clean-fast-safe beverage
- ❏ I went on a walk
- ❏ I imagined my body tapping into my fat stores for fuel
- ❏ _____
  _____
- ❏ _____
  _____
- ❏ _____
  _____

EATING WINDOW CHECK-IN

Eating Window Length Goal: _____ hours
Actual Eating Window Length: _____ hours

How do I feel about today's eating window?

_____
_____
_____
_____
_____
_____
_____
_____
_____

What went well? Was there anything that I struggled with during my eating window? _____

_____

_____

_____

_____

_____

_____

_____

_____

_____

_____

TODAY'S NSVS, OR NON-SCALE VICTORIES

One of the most powerful things we can do is acknowledge our Non-Scale Victories (NSVs). These can be physical (*pain reduction, better energy, mental clarity, etc.*) or emotional (*freedom around food, confidence, etc.*).

What were today's NSVs? _____

_____

_____

_____

_____

_____

_____

_____

_____

REFLECTIONS

Today, I listened to my body when I: _____

_____

_____

_____

_____

_____

_____

_____

Today's *AHA!* moment(s): _____

_____

_____

_____

Something that is on my mind: _____

_____

_____

_____

_____

PREPARING FOR SUCCESS

Goal(s) and/or strategies for tomorrow: _____

_____

_____

_____

_____

WEEK 3 PLAN

Which approach did you choose for last week?

☐ The *Easy Does It* Approach (ten-hour window, low-carb ease-in breakfast or early lunch, low-carb ease-in snack, plus a regular dinner)

☐ The *Steady Build* Approach (seven-hour window, including lunch and dinner)

☐ The *Rip Off the Band-Aid* Approach (six-hour window, including lunch *or* snack, and dinner)

How did it go?

☐ It was too easy! I think I can ramp it up this week.

☐ It was JUST RIGHT. Not too hard, not too easy.

☐ It was too much for me. I am going to scale it back this week.

Which approach will you follow for week 3?

☐ The *Easy Does It* Approach (eight-hour window, including a low-carb ease-in lunch, plus a regular dinner)

☐ The *Steady Build* Approach (six-hour window, including lunch *or* snack, and dinner)

☐ The *Rip Off the Band-Aid* Approach (five-hour window, including lunch *or* snack, and dinner)

DAY 15: GO AT YOUR OWN PACE— *MORE* ISN'T ALWAYS "BETTER"

Today's Date: _____

PLANNING FOR A SUCCESSFUL DAY 15

Today, I am following

❑ The *Easy Does It* Approach (eight-hour window, including a low-carb ease-in lunch, plus a regular dinner)
❑ The *Steady Build* Approach (six-hour window, including lunch *or* snack, and dinner)
❑ The *Rip Off the Band-Aid* Approach (five-hour window, including lunch *or* snack, and dinner)

My personal goal(s) for today: _____

_____

_____

_____

_____

15

Daily Lesson from Gin: Go at your own pace—MORE isn't always "better."

You are just past the halfway point of your FAST Start, and that's something to celebrate! As you begin week 3, take time to consciously reflect on how you're doing.

Before flipping the page to day 15, you planned how you would approach this coming week, and perhaps you decided you wanted to ramp things up. In theory, there is nothing wrong with that. In practice, however, it may be a different story.

"Just Do It!"

You probably recognize the Nike slogan; most of us have grown up hearing it. At some point, many of us internalized the message that our goal should always be to push harder, harder, and then harder still. If you aren't pushing yourself to your limits, you should push yourself *more*.

"No Pain, No Gain!"

I'm sure that saying is also familiar to you.

I want to teach you a different way to think about things.

When we try to do more than our bodies (or minds) are ready for, that can often lead to crashing and burning. Never forget the analogy I gave on day 9. If you want to run a 5K but you've been sedentary for years, you wouldn't get up and go run a 5K on day 1. Your body isn't ready for that. Instead, you might choose a couch-to-5K program that would allow you to build up your endurance from day to day, until one day you are able to run the entire 5K without stopping.

As you move into week 3, remember that your goal is to live an intermittent fasting lifestyle, and the 28-Day FAST Start is the time that your body is learning to do something new. Before you started, you made a commitment to yourself that you would not quit.

Part of keeping that promise to yourself is making sure that what you are doing is sustainable.

Trying to do more than your body is ready for is not sustainable.

If you need to adjust your approach at any time, do it. Remind yourself: MORE isn't always better.

DAILY INSPIRATION SPOTLIGHT:
Mary Lou Reece, Dallas, Texas
Intermittent Fasting Stories guest, episode 72

How long has she been an intermittent faster? *Between three and four years.*

My daughter was told by her ob-gyn about IF four years ago and began to fast to help with mild PCOS. She was a bit afraid to tell me about it, thinking I wouldn't like it, but as soon as she told me, I thought, Hmmm I might be able to do that. I have never been a fad dieter or done a named diet. Twice in my life I'd lost 50 pounds on just calorie restriction. But calorie-restriction weight loss was the hardest thing ever! I thought about food all the time. I even dreamed about food! But I'm an all-or-nothing kind of person. So, if I tell myself I can't ever eat any particular thing, I am doomed, because as soon as I do, all is lost, and I'm done. When I heard about IF, I thought that not eating and then eating what I wanted in a time frame had a LOT of appeal. I really had in my mind that if I could ever just get to 145, that would be ideal. I would not even dream about weighing less than that (amazingly, I'm now 20 pounds under that dream). I am five foot four (almost). The first pounds melted away, but mostly the inches around my waist melted before the pounds. I've stayed within a 4-pound margin ever since. I did not change my eating pattern really, although I'm looser with how many two-meal days and treats I have now. But I have never really had to deny myself anything. I was able to get off my digestive meds within a month—A MONTH—of intermittent fasting! I'd been trying to get off for a few years

15

with no success. I do find I like to eat better food now, and I crave salads like I never did before. One more thing—for most of these almost four years, I have ridden a bike fifteen to twenty-five miles, four or five times a week (and I'm no spring chicken). I can do that at twenty to twenty-five hours fasted. My body knows how to make energy. The body is amazing. I'm so blessed. And I'm so thankful for this way of eating and Gin's persistent work toward understanding and clear communication to make it accessible!

ADVICE FROM MARY LOU

One: Read the dang book, either one (Delay, Don't Deny or Fast. Feast. Repeat.). I've never had a friend be successful long term if they didn't actually read the book to understand the process. It's an easy read, very accessible. Just Do It! Two: Don't obsess! Not everything that happens to your body in that first six months is because of fasting. Give your body time to adapt.

YOU HAVE ALL THE TOOLS YOU NEED TO SUCCEED.
ENJOY YOUR DAY! YOU'VE GOT THIS.

HOW DID IT GO?
IT'S TIME TO REFLECT ON DAY 15.

TODAY (CHECK ALL THAT APPLY):

❏ I fasted clean (plain water, unflavored sparkling water, black unflavored coffee, plain tea)
❏ During the fast, I took time to reflect on the positive changes happening in my body
❏ Within my eating window, I ate until I was satisfied, and then I stopped
❏ I honored my "I've had enough" signals
❏ I stayed off the scale

FAST CHECK-IN

Rate the difficulty of today's fast on a scale from 1 to 10 (circle one):

1　2　3　4　5　6　7　8　9　**10**

(Today was easy! I sailed right through it.)　　(Today was HARD! I struggled.)

During today's fast, I felt _____
_____
_____
_____
_____
_____

(*examples: exhilarated, hopeful, hungry, uncomfortable, bored, etc.*)

I used these strategies to manage my feelings today (check all that apply and add your own):

- ❏ I remembered my *why*
- ❏ I stayed busy
- ❏ I enjoyed a clean-fast-safe beverage
- ❏ I went on a walk
- ❏ I imagined my body tapping into my fat stores for fuel
- ❏ _____
  _____
- ❏ _____
  _____
- ❏ _____
  _____

EATING WINDOW CHECK-IN

Eating Window Length Goal: _____ hours
Actual Eating Window Length: _____ hours

How do I feel about today's eating window?
_____
_____
_____
_____
_____
_____
_____
_____
_____

What went well? Was there anything that I struggled with during my eating window? _____

_____

_____

_____

_____

_____

_____

_____

_____

_____

_____

TODAY'S NSVS, OR NON-SCALE VICTORIES

One of the most powerful things we can do is acknowledge our Non-Scale Victories (NSVs). These can be physical (*pain reduction, better energy, mental clarity, etc.*) or emotional (*freedom around food, confidence, etc.*).

What were today's NSVs? _____

_____

_____

_____

_____

_____

_____

_____

_____

_____

REFLECTIONS

Today, I listened to my body when I: _____

_____

_____

_____

_____

_____

_____

_____

Today's *AHA!* moment(s): _____

_____

_____

_____

Something that is on my mind: _____

_____

_____

_____

PREPARING FOR SUCCESS

Goal(s) and/or strategies for tomorrow: _____

_____

_____

_____

_____

DAY 16: DEALING WITH HUNGER

Today's Date: _____

PLANNING FOR A SUCCESSFUL DAY 16

Today, I am following

- ❏ The *Easy Does It* Approach (eight-hour window, including a low-carb ease-in lunch, plus a regular dinner)
- ❏ The *Steady Build* Approach (six-hour window, including lunch *or* snack, and dinner)
- ❏ The *Rip Off the Band-Aid* Approach (five-hour window, including lunch *or* snack, and dinner)

My personal goal(s) for today: _____

_____

_____

_____

_____

16

Daily Lesson from Gin: Dealing with hunger.

You may have found my work through my podcast, *Intermittent Fasting Stories*. A lot of people have found inspiration through the hundreds of stories that have been shared by all types of IFers over the years.

Even though we have hundreds of stories, each is unique. On the other hand, there are common threads that run between all of them. Listening to the stories is like meeting a new friend in every episode.

Still, listeners may come away with this thought after listening:

Those podcast guests make it sound so easy. It isn't always easy for me!

While many guests (and I) may make it sound like living an intermittent fasting lifestyle is always easy, that isn't always the case. Some days will be harder than others, especially during your FAST Start. But, as I explained on day 13, you *can* do hard things. And even the hardest days as an IFer are easier in comparison to the years I spent on the diet train. Dieting was so much harder than simply delaying my eating window for the day.

Podcast listeners may also get the impression that if you're an intermittent faster, you should never be "hungry" during the day. If they feel hungry, they think it means they are doing something wrong.

I have good news for you, and also some bad news. Let's start with the bad news and get that out of the way.

I have been living an intermittent fasting lifestyle consistently since 2014, and I still get hunger during the fast every single day. In fact, as I typed that sentence, I experienced a mild wave of hunger. (The mind is a powerful thing! Just thinking about hunger brought it on.)

So, the bad news is that being an intermittent faster doesn't mean that you'll have a life free of hunger.

The good news is that hunger is not an emergency, and it is actually a fleeting sensation.

Before I was an intermittent faster, I had the impression that hunger would build and build until it got so bad that I would faint or not be able to go on without food. Somehow, commercials and ads have taught us that hunger is some sort of crisis that must be avoided at all costs. For best results, carry snacks with you at all times, and if you feel even the *slightest hint of hunger*, the only way to handle it is to put some food into your body *immediately*.

Well, that's great for the snack manufacturers. But it isn't great for our bodies. When you are constantly putting snacks and meals into your body, you keep your insulin levels high. You're in constant storage mode.

We don't want to be in constant storage mode. That is why we end up overweight and metabolically unhealthy. Instead, we need to give our bodies time to do the important cellular housekeeping (hello, autophagy!), and we also want our bodies to use the glucose that got stored away from our last meal and also to venture into our fat stores for some of the fuel that may have been stashed away for years, just waiting to be needed.

On day 9, I explained what happens when we train our bodies to flip our metabolic switch. After we have depleted liver glycogen sufficiently, there's no more quick fuel available. What's a body to do? Hello, fat-burning superpower! Hello, ketosis!

16

How do we know that is happening? Wouldn't it be nice if we came equipped with a fuel tank that let us know?

Well, we kinda do. Let me explain.

Recently, I've been wearing a CGM, which is a *continuous glucose monitor*. A CGM gives you tremendous insight into what your blood glucose is doing throughout the day so you'll know how your body responds to the foods you eat, among other things.

So, what does a CGM have to do with hunger during fasting? Thanks to the CGM, I realized something fascinating that I wasn't expecting to see. When I have the most persistent hunger wave during my fast, that is when my blood glucose is heading gently downward. My body begins sending me gentle "You could eat now if you want to!" messages.

When I don't send down a quick source of fuel in response to my body's gentle urgings, I picture my body flipping that metabolic switch and entering ketosis. I'm able to chug along happily, well fueled until it's time to open my window.

I actually welcome that mild hunger each day now. It's physical confirmation that my body is flipping the metabolic switch and entering the deep-cleaning phase for the day. Maybe I feel uncomfortable for a few minutes, but it goes away, and then I feel great.

NOTE: Do you need to wear a CGM to live an intermittent fasting lifestyle? The answer is NO. I have been living an IF lifestyle for years and only recently began using a CGM. While wearing a CGM has gently prodded me to focus on higher-quality foods within my eating window, we don't need a CGM to tell us that real food is always going to be better for our bodies than ultra-processed foods, and we also don't need a CGM to let us know our bodies are flipping the metabolic switch.

Here's something else that is important to understand about hunger. Back when I was eating all day long and following conventional dietary advice to eat three meals plus multiple snacks, I actually experienced a lot more hunger throughout the day than I do now. Every time I had those mild hunger waves, I fed them. That led to my blood sugar going up (after eating) and then back down (which brought on yet another hunger wave). That was a no-win situation, because every time I ate, I was setting myself up to be hungry again as soon as my body had dealt with the food I had eaten. Since I was trapped in storage mode, my body happily stored it all away for later, and because I always added more fuel every time I felt mild hunger, "later" never came.

I also want to make one important distinction about hunger: often, you may confuse "hunger" with other sensations. A growling stomach is the mechanical action of an empty stomach, and it doesn't mean you need to eat. Sometimes, we may be bored, and food starts calling our names. That isn't true hunger, either.

If you feel shaky or nauseous, however, that is an indication that you *do* need to eat. Don't try to push through those sensations.

During the FAST Start, when your body isn't yet skilled at flipping the metabolic switch, you may find you have those moments where you actually do feel shaky or nauseous and need to go ahead and open your window for the day. Don't feel like you're a failure. Never forget that your body is learning how to do something new. Teaching your body to become metabolically flexible is a process.

16

Once your body adapts and is able to flip the metabolic switch, you shouldn't have that issue. If you do continue to get shaky day after day, that's when you need to examine your fast carefully and make sure it's truly squeaky clean. I can't tell you how many times I've heard IFers talk about how their hunger never gets better, and when we dig in, we realize they are drinking something that breaks their fast, like an herbal tea or a bottled coffee product with additives (such as citric acid or natural flavors). Those fast-breakers cause an insulin response (the CPIR I explained on day 1), and insulin does its job and lowers blood sugar, leading to the shakiness and nausea. As I said, when that happens, go ahead and eat.

Here's something else that is important to understand: you may be wondering what happens when you lose all the weight you want to lose. Does your body just keep burning more and more fat each day, until you end up at an unhealthy low weight? The answer to that question is no.

Our bodies have one goal: they want us to survive. For that reason, they will do anything possible to keep you from ending up at a lower weight than is healthy for your body. One of the first things that happens is that you get an increased appetite to keep you from losing too much weight.

I'm in maintenance now (and not actively gaining or losing fat), so I maintain a balance between the fuel I put in during my eating window and the fuel my body takes out during the fast. When we reach this point of homeostasis, "appetite correction" drives us to eat a bit more within our eating windows so we don't lose more weight than our bodies want us to lose. I'll talk more about that concept in tomorrow's lesson.

DAILY INSPIRATION SPOTLIGHT:
Daniel Hale, Monmouth Junction, New Jersey
Intermittent Fasting Stories guest, episode 102

How long has he been an intermittent faster? *Between three and four years.*

I started fasting in the fall of 2019 just one day a week as an experiment. After a few months, I found that I felt best on that day, so I began fasting daily. I followed the 16:8 protocol, which led to 18:6, which then led to a 20:4 and finally OMAD (one meal a day). The fasting, combined with eating whole foods cooked from home, helped me lose 130 pounds. This was all shared on the podcast, which was in the spring of 2020. In the almost three years since the podcast, I have continued my fasting journey. During that first year, I religiously tracked my fasts each day. It was great motivation to build long streaks and helped keep me on track. After a while, I decided to stop tracking pretty much everything. I had kept off the weight for over a year and a half at this point and felt that I had everything on autopilot. During this time, I continued to fast daily and did not need to track, as fasting is just what made me feel best. My work schedule changed a bit, which forced me to experiment with different windows. I always liked waiting until the end of the evening when everything was done for the day before I would eat. But now I was working so late that it did not seem like an option. I experimented with earlier-morning windows and midafternoon windows. I found myself still wanting to eat when I would get home from work even if I had eaten enough during my window. I then found a good balance for a while eating a small meal in the late morning and then another meal at night. To this day, I continue to experiment with various types of fasting due to my ever-changing work schedule. Recently, I have gone back to OMAD and tracking my fasts with an app. Specifically for the days that I was eating my meal in an earlier window, I wanted some accountability to keep me from snacking late at night. Keep in mind that a fasting journey is definitely not linear and is always evolving. It is very easy for me to switch back and forth between various fasting protocols due to all the experience I have gained. I am able to easily go

16

long periods of time without eating regardless of when I choose to eat. I enjoy this freedom around food that I had not had in my previous, non-fasting life!

ADVICE FROM DANIEL

Please understand that this is a lifelong journey, and be willing to experiment. Your life will change, and you can also change the way you fast to adapt. There is not one way to do it, and through experimentation and giving yourself grace when things don't go as planned, you can find what works for you.

**YOU HAVE ALL THE TOOLS YOU NEED TO SUCCEED.
ENJOY YOUR DAY! YOU'VE GOT THIS.**

HOW DID IT GO?
IT'S TIME TO REFLECT ON DAY 16.

TODAY (CHECK ALL THAT APPLY):

❑ I fasted clean (plain water, unflavored sparkling water, black unflavored coffee, plain tea)

❑ During the fast, I took time to reflect on the positive changes happening in my body

❑ Within my eating window, I ate until I was satisfied, and then I stopped

❑ I honored my "I've had enough" signals

❑ I stayed off the scale

FAST CHECK-IN

Rate the difficulty of today's fast on a scale from 1 to 10 (circle one):

1   2   3   4   5   6   7   8   9   **10**

(Today was easy! I sailed right through it.)   (Today was HARD! I struggled.)

During today's fast, I felt _____

_____

_____

_____

_____

_____

(*examples: exhilarated, hopeful, hungry, uncomfortable, bored, etc.*)

I used these strategies to manage my feelings today (check all that apply and add your own):

- ❏ I remembered my *why*
- ❏ I stayed busy
- ❏ I enjoyed a clean-fast-safe beverage
- ❏ I went on a walk
- ❏ I imagined my body tapping into my fat stores for fuel
- ❏ _____
  _____
- ❏ _____
  _____
- ❏ _____
  _____

EATING WINDOW CHECK-IN

Eating Window Length Goal: _____ hours
Actual Eating Window Length: _____ hours

How do I feel about today's eating window?

_____
_____
_____
_____
_____
_____
_____
_____
_____

What went well? Was there anything that I struggled with during my eating window? _____

_____

_____

_____

_____

_____

_____

_____

_____

_____

_____

TODAY'S NSVS, OR NON-SCALE VICTORIES

One of the most powerful things we can do is acknowledge our Non-Scale Victories (NSVs). These can be physical (*pain reduction, better energy, mental clarity, etc.*) or emotional (*freedom around food, confidence, etc.*).

What were today's NSVs? _____

_____

_____

_____

_____

_____

_____

_____

_____

_____

REFLECTIONS

Today, I listened to my body when I: _____

_____

_____

_____

_____

_____

_____

_____

Today's *AHA!* moment(s): _____

_____

_____

_____

Something that is on my mind: _____

_____

_____

_____

PREPARING FOR SUCCESS

Goal(s) and/or strategies for tomorrow: _____

_____

_____

_____

_____

DAY 17: CONNECTING WITH OUR SATIETY SIGNALS: WHAT IS APPETITE CORRECTION?

Today's Date: _____

PLANNING FOR A SUCCESSFUL DAY 17

Today, I am following

❏ The *Easy Does It* Approach (eight-hour window, including a low-carb ease-in lunch, plus a regular dinner)
❏ The *Steady Build* Approach (six-hour window, including lunch *or* snack, and dinner)
❏ The *Rip Off the Band-Aid* Approach (five-hour window, including lunch *or* snack, and dinner)

17

My personal goal(s) for today: _____
_____
_____
_____
_____
_____

Daily Lesson from Gin: Connecting with our satiety signals: what is appetite correction?

The term *appetite correction* was coined by Dr. Bert Herring in his book called *AC: The Power of Appetite Correction.* It's a brilliant term, and I am so glad that he put it out into the world.

What does appetite correction mean? It means that you

are back in tune with your body's appetite control center: the appestat. When you experience appetite correction, you don't need to count calories to know when you have had enough to eat . . . your body sends you the "stop eating" signals, *and* you can hear them. (Of course, you still have to *listen* to these signals. It's possible to override them and keep eating. If that happens, you'll likely wish you had stopped when you first got the signal. We have all been there, and after you feel that *"Oops! I ate too much!"* feeling a few times, you learn to listen more closely.)

What exactly is the appestat? Within the hypothalamus region of our brains, we have both a "satiety center" and a "feeding center," which make up our appestat.

How does the appestat work? In theory, it works like your home's thermostat. When your body senses that you need to eat more food, it cranks up your hunger hormones and turns down your satiety hormones. The result is that you are hormonally driven to eat more food and don't feel easily satisfied. In contrast, when your body decides you have had enough, it can decrease your hunger hormones and increase satiety hormones so that you stop eating.

If you've ever spent time with a newborn baby, you have seen this in action. When a baby is hungry, no one can rest until that baby is fed! How does the baby *know* it is hungry? After all, the baby isn't counting calories. It's the appestat!

On the flip side, once a baby has had enough to eat, there is no way you are going to convince him to take in another drop. I remember trying to feed my older son, and he had this thing he did with his lips that was a clear signal that he was *not* going to have any more, no matter how much I tried to get him to. How did he *know* he had enough? Again, it's the appestat!

It's probably been a long time since you were able to hear your hunger and satiety signals as well as a newborn baby. Keep one thing in mind: some people *never lose* their connections with their appestats! These are your friends and family members who have remained lean for their whole lives . . . the ones who you watch with amazement at holiday gatherings as they put down their forks with cake *still left on the plate*. We think of those people as "naturally thin," and my husband is one of them. He *always* knew how to stop eating when he had enough food, and he couldn't understand why I was unable to just do the same.

Somehow, along the way, however, the rest of us lose touch with the signals from our hunger and satiety hormones.

The good news is that intermittent fasting helps us reconnect with those signals over time.

Here's something to also understand about appetite correction: it works both ways! Sometimes, IFers think that appetite correction only means that we get full quickly and find it easy to stop when satisfied. That's part of it, but not the end of the story! Some days, you'll have an *increased* appetite. Listen to your body when that happens! Increased hunger on some days is also a feature of appetite correction. Once we understand this fact, we can be a lot easier on ourselves when we have a hungrier day. It's not just because you are *weak* or *bad* or a glutton. No, hormones are powerful things, and it's hard to resist their mighty signals! Some days you simply need to eat more food.

When we learn to listen to our bodies, we don't need to

count calories or track macros. We trust our satiety (and hunger) signals, and we *stop when satisfied* (or eat more when we need to).

It's so important to never forget this one fact, though: when you are trying to lose weight, the amount you eat *does* matter. Your goal is to *stop when satisfied*, and not to keep eating more just because your window is still open. You want to *stop when satisfied*, not overly full. You know that Thanksgiving Day overstuffed feeling? That's how you feel when you eat too much. We don't want to get to that point. *Stop when satisfied.*

> **I keep repeating those words:**
> **Stop when satisfied.**

This can be a difficult thing for new intermittent fasters who are trying to embrace the concept of appetite correction but aren't there yet.

Maybe you are not in tune with your satiety signals yet, and it's going to take a while longer for you. That's totally to be expected during the adjustment period. If you remember the lessons from day 9 and day 11, I explained that during the FAST Start, your body isn't well fueled during your daily fast because it hasn't yet learned to flip the metabolic switch. Hang in there! It will get better.

Eventually, you will finally be able to *hear* your satiety signals, but you still may not be good at *listening* to them. Learning to both hear and obey your "I've had enough" signals is where the power lies.

Another piece of the puzzle is that some of our eating and drinking habits may interfere with us connecting to our satiety signals. Ultra-processed foods keep us from feeling satisfied because they don't provide the nutrients our bodies are looking for. Alcohol can also have a negative impact on our ability to hear the "I've had enough" signals. If you find you are struggling with stopping when satisfied, one of the most powerful things you can do is focus on high-quality foods—real food—and also you may want to delay alcohol for a time, or simply cut back on intake.

EXTRA CREDIT READING

Read chapter 16 of *Fast. Feast. Repeat.* for a deeper dive into appetite correction. Chapters 15 and 17 of *Fast. Feast. Repeat.* will also help you understand the importance of food quality when it comes to tuning into your appetite correction.

17

DAILY INSPIRATION SPOTLIGHT:
Michelle Williams, St. Louis, Missouri
Intermittent Fasting Stories guest, episode 126 and episode 220

How long has she been an intermittent faster? *Over five years.*

I stumbled upon intermittent fasting in 2013 after trying every diet known to mankind and being unsuccessful at keeping the weight off. I decided to start listening to my body and only eating one meal a day. I was never hungry in the morning, and when I ate midday, I noticed that I became extremely tired and unproductive, and I was even hungrier within a couple of hours. When I initially started eating one meal a day, I was just trying to reduce calories and thought that is why I lost over forty pounds within a couple of months. Friends and family eventually convinced me that eating one meal a day was unhealthy and that I was starving myself. I resumed eating multiple meals a day, and the weight piled back on. My weight continued to climb for the next several years. I remembered that the only thing that had worked for me in the past was eating one meal a day. I started researching if eating one meal a day was healthy. That is when I came across the term intermittent fasting. When I started researching intermittent fasting more, I came across Jason Fung's work and of course Gin Stephens's book Delay, Don't Deny. I finally had the science behind why eating one meal a day had worked so well for me back in 2013. I went on to lose over seventy pounds. Then the pandemic happened and many other life-altering events, such as being diagnosed with a mental health condition and helping my son through a tragic event. I was placed on medication for several months and started eating multiple meals a day. I also began to use food as a coping mechanism again to deal with stress and depression. I gained back most of the weight that I had lost. Through all of this, I still had intermittent fasting as a tool in my toolbox. After my mental health issue was stabilized and my son overcame his ordeal, I resumed intermittent fasting, and to date, I have lost almost all the weight that I regained. I became a certified holistic wellness coach. I published a book called Elegant Elevation: Shattering Through the Glass Ceiling to Become the Best Version of You. I have also started a Facebook group called Elegant Elevation Intermittent Fasting Group where I coach other people on intermittent fasting. I truly thank Gin for being a trailblazer in this global fight against weight gain and obesity and for helping us learn to naturally heal our bodies. Intermittent fasting also had a positive impact in so many other areas of my life.

ADVICE FROM MICHELLE

My advice to anyone new or returning to intermittent fasting is to be patient, trust the process of intermittent fasting, and give yourself grace. I would also encourage you to educate yourself on the benefits of intermittent fasting from reputable sources such as Jason Fung and Gin Stephens. Research and understand bio-individuality, listen to your body, and find the foods that work best for you. Most importantly, identify and remember your why. Identify why you may be overeating in the first place, deal with those issues, and remember why you want to live a healthier lifestyle. You can do this, and you are worth it!

17

**YOU HAVE ALL THE TOOLS YOU NEED TO SUCCEED.
ENJOY YOUR DAY! YOU'VE GOT THIS.**

HOW DID IT GO?
IT'S TIME TO REFLECT ON DAY 17.

TODAY (CHECK ALL THAT APPLY):

❏ I fasted clean (plain water, unflavored sparkling water, black unflavored coffee, plain tea)

❏ During the fast, I took time to reflect on the positive changes happening in my body

❏ Within my eating window, I ate until I was satisfied, and then I stopped

❏ I honored my "I've had enough" signals

❏ I stayed off the scale

FAST CHECK-IN

Rate the difficulty of today's fast on a scale from 1 to 10 (circle one):

1　2　3　4　5　6　7　8　9　**10**

(Today was easy! I sailed right through it.)　　(Today was HARD! I struggled.)

During today's fast, I felt _____

_____

_____

_____

_____

_____

(*examples: exhilarated, hopeful, hungry, uncomfortable, bored, etc.*)

I used these strategies to manage my feelings today (check all that apply and add your own):

- ❑ I remembered my *why*
- ❑ I stayed busy
- ❑ I enjoyed a clean-fast-safe beverage
- ❑ I went on a walk
- ❑ I imagined my body tapping into my fat stores for fuel
- ❑ _____
  _____
- ❑ _____
  _____
- ❑ _____
  _____

EATING WINDOW CHECK-IN

Eating Window Length Goal: _____ hours
Actual Eating Window Length: _____ hours

How do I feel about today's eating window?

_____
_____
_____
_____
_____
_____
_____
_____
_____
_____

What went well? Was there anything that I struggled with during my eating window? _____

_____

_____

_____

_____

_____

_____

_____

_____

_____

TODAY'S NSVS, OR NON-SCALE VICTORIES

One of the most powerful things we can do is acknowledge our Non-Scale Victories (NSVs). These can be physical (*pain reduction, better energy, mental clarity, etc.*) or emotional (*freedom around food, confidence, etc.*).

What were today's NSVs? _____

_____

_____

_____

_____

_____

_____

_____

_____

REFLECTIONS

Today, I listened to my body when I: _____

_____

_____

_____

_____

_____

_____

_____

Today's *AHA!* moment(s): _____

_____

_____

_____

_____

Something that is on my mind: _____

_____

_____

_____

_____

PREPARING FOR SUCCESS

Goal(s) and/or strategies for tomorrow: _____

_____

_____

_____

_____

_____

DAY 18: GET UP AND *MOVE*!

Today's Date: _____

PLANNING FOR A SUCCESSFUL DAY 18

Today, I am following

- ❏ The *Easy Does It* Approach (eight-hour window, including a low-carb ease-in lunch, plus a regular dinner)
- ❏ The *Steady Build* Approach (six-hour window, including lunch *or* snack, and dinner)
- ❏ The *Rip Off the Band-Aid* Approach (five-hour window, including lunch *or* snack, and dinner)

My personal goal(s) for today: _____

_____

_____

_____

_____

Daily Lesson from Gin: Get up and MOVE!

You may have already figured this out by now, but it can be hard to do intense exercise in the fasted state during the adjustment period. Many new IFers who are used to having an exercise regimen are surprised to discover that they don't have the stamina or endurance they used to have prior to IF.

The good news is that it's temporary.

As you already have learned, when you initially begin your IF lifestyle, your body is not yet skilled at fueling itself from stored fat. If you try to work out and your body can't find the fuel it needs, you're going to struggle through what normally might be easy for you.

Once your body adapts to IF, however, you'll have plenty of energy for fasted workouts. Before that happens, be patient with your body, and you'll likely do better to take a gentler approach for now.

It's really important to remember that the way you feel during the adjustment period is not how you're going to feel forever.

Now that you're eighteen days into your FAST Start, you may be starting to feel a little worse (meaning that you are on your way to flipping your metabolic switch), or maybe you've already progressed through that "feeling worse" phase and you're starting to feel better.

Either way, now is a great time to add some purposeful movement to your day. Adding gentle movement such as walking can help your body deplete your glycogen stores, which will speed up your physical adaptation. Hooray for that!

In addition to speeding up your body's adaptation, adding movement is a great strategy to use at your previous meal or snack times throughout your day. Instead of sitting around and feeling sad that you aren't eating, get moving and tell your body: "Eat my fat!"

I always smile when I am doing some sort of activity during my fast and tell my body to eat fat. It's a powerful mental image.

18

EXTRA CREDIT READING

I am sure you have many more questions about exercise and fasting, and I've got you covered! Read chapter 21 of *Fast. Feast. Repeat.* for an in-depth discussion of all things IF and exercise. In that chapter, I explain important concepts, such as why you don't need to fuel up directly before, during, or after a workout (thank you to both our fat-burning superpower and autophagy!).

DAILY INSPIRATION SPOTLIGHT:
Barbara DeLeo, Marlborough, New Zealand
Intermittent Fasting Stories guest, episode 169

How long has she been an intermittent faster? *Between three and four years.*

As I was getting closer and closer to fifty, I was finding it harder and harder to maintain my weight. I'd always had to watch what I ate and was resigned to the fact that I would always be the one who had to say no to the ice cream or the carrot cake. I'd accepted that my future was going to be walking farther and lifting more often, just to stay the same. In an effort to slow the inevitable, I tried keto, then Noom, then low sugar, then Paleo, but to my horror, the scale began to inch up. I'd read about fasting while I was failing miserably at keto and had thought how ridiculously difficult that would be—I mean, eating less and less was hard enough, but to eat nothing at all?! When my husband returned from a trip to see friends in Australia and mentioned they were fasting, he quietly suggested we try it.

That was August of 2019, and we have both fasted every day since. I read Delay, Don't Deny *in one sitting and began clean fasting straightaway. We did 16:8 for a week or two, then quickly moved through 18:6 and settled at 19:5. We had four teenagers at home and wanted to still eat dinner as a family, so that worked well. We'd both open our window about 2:00 p.m. and close by 7:00 p.m. My weight loss was slow, but I eventually lost five kilograms (eleven pounds) and my husband lost ten kilograms (twenty-two pounds), but the biggest change was in what I was eating. I finally felt satisfied when I had finished a meal. I could eat ice cream and cake again in moderation, but most of the time, I just ate what I felt like—delicious, whole food. We are now into our fourth year of fasting, and we've changed our protocol again. Our kids are all away at university, and we both work from home so have a similar schedule. Sunday–Thursday we open our window at about 1:30 p.m. with a salad and then have our main meal, which is usually fish or eggs with lots of different vegetables (I'm vegetarian), and then we'll have fruit and yogurt, maybe a dessert, or some nuts and cheese, then we'll close by 3:30 p.m. Friday and Saturday, we'll open a little later and extend our window until about 7:00 or 8:00 p.m. so we can have a drink or dinner with friends. We only drink black coffee, green tea, or water during the fast. We are both the most fit and healthy we've ever been. I walk the dog and do reformer Pilates and lift weights a couple of times a week, but I'm much more relaxed about it and don't worry if I miss a few days. In the five years before fasting, I'd had ten basal and squamous cell skin cancers removed, and since fasting, I've had none. The thing about fasting is that it is one hundred times easier than spending every day restricting what you eat, just to stay the same. I sleep better, my body shape has completely changed, and I've found the pleasure in food again.*

ADVICE FROM BARBARA

IF is EASY. No, it really is. If you take your time becoming fat adapted (slowly increasing the length of your fast), if you truly fast clean, and if you eat mostly a well-balanced, nutritionally dense diet in your eating window, IF is easy enough to do forever. It's not a lie to say that I have eaten more ice cream in the last three years than I had in the twenty years before fasting. The FREEDOM of that, knowing I can eat any type of food I want in my eating window, is a game changer. And because IF is so easy, it follows that consistency is easy and therefore new habits are easy as well. I drink way more water now that I'm fasting. Before fasting, I would have a glass or two of wine every night, but as I close my window at 3:30 p.m. most days, I only drink a couple of days a week, so I've cut down hugely on my alcohol consumption. I am so grateful to have found IF and to live this lifestyle every day.

**YOU HAVE ALL THE TOOLS YOU NEED TO SUCCEED.
ENJOY YOUR DAY! YOU'VE GOT THIS.**

HOW DID IT GO?
IT'S TIME TO REFLECT ON DAY 18.

TODAY (CHECK ALL THAT APPLY):

- ❏ I fasted clean (plain water, unflavored sparkling water, black unflavored coffee, plain tea)
- ❏ During the fast, I took time to reflect on the positive changes happening in my body
- ❏ Within my eating window, I ate until I was satisfied, and then I stopped
- ❏ I honored my "I've had enough" signals
- ❏ I stayed off the scale

FAST CHECK-IN

Rate the difficulty of today's fast on a scale from 1 to 10 (circle one):

1　2　3　4　5　6　7　8　9　**10**

(Today was easy! I sailed right through it.)　　(Today was HARD! I struggled.)

During today's fast, I felt _____

_____

_____

_____

_____

_____

(*examples: exhilarated, hopeful, hungry, uncomfortable, bored, etc.*)

I used these strategies to manage my feelings today (check all that apply and add your own):

- ❏ I remembered my *why*
- ❏ I stayed busy
- ❏ I enjoyed a clean-fast-safe beverage
- ❏ I went on a walk
- ❏ I imagined my body tapping into my fat stores for fuel
- ❏ _____
  _____
- ❏ _____
  _____
- ❏ _____
  _____

EATING WINDOW CHECK-IN

Eating Window Length Goal: _____ hours
Actual Eating Window Length: _____ hours

How do I feel about today's eating window?

_____
_____
_____
_____
_____
_____
_____
_____
_____

What went well? Was there anything that I struggled with during my eating window? _____

_____

_____

_____

_____

_____

_____

_____

_____

_____

TODAY'S NSVS, OR NON-SCALE VICTORIES

One of the most powerful things we can do is acknowledge our Non-Scale Victories (NSVs). These can be physical (*pain reduction, better energy, mental clarity, etc.*) or emotional (*freedom around food, confidence, etc.*).

What were today's NSVs? _____

_____

_____

_____

_____

_____

_____

_____

_____

REFLECTIONS

Today, I listened to my body when I: _____

_____

_____

_____

_____

_____

_____

_____

_____

Today's *AHA!* moment(s): _____

_____

_____

_____

_____

Something that is on my mind: _____

_____

_____

_____

_____

PREPARING FOR SUCCESS

Goal(s) and/or strategies for tomorrow: _____

_____

_____

_____

_____

DAY 19: THE SCIENCE OF HABIT CREATION— *KEEP GOING!*

Today's Date: _____

PLANNING FOR A SUCCESSFUL DAY 19

Today, I am following

19

❏ The *Easy Does It* Approach (eight-hour window, including a low-carb ease-in lunch, plus a regular dinner)
❏ The *Steady Build* Approach (six-hour window, including lunch *or* snack, and dinner)
❏ The *Rip Off the Band-Aid* Approach (five-hour window, including lunch *or* snack, and dinner)

My personal goal(s) for today: _____

_____

_____

_____

_____

Daily Lesson from Gin: The science of habit creation— *KEEP GOING!*

In the summer of 2020, I'll never forget the exciting day that I learned my book *Fast. Feast. Repeat.* had made the *New York Times* Best Sellers List. That was such a thrilling moment, and I will never take it for granted. I'm grateful for every person who had a part in making it happen.

I was at the beach that day, and my beach read just happened to be *Atomic Habits* by James Clear. Here's what felt surreal: I was reading *Atomic Habits*, which was #3 on the *New York Times* Best Sellers List that week, and guess what was #4? Yep. *Fast. Feast. Repeat. Atomic Habits* was my next-door book-neighbor. Joanna Gaines was at #2 with her latest *Magnolia Table* book. I'll always feel a kinship with those two books, like we are all book-friends from our time together on the list (I have also watched every single episode of *Fixer Upper*, and I think every viewer falls in love with Joanna and her husband, Chip, after watching).

You may be wondering why I just told you that story, and it has to do with today's lesson: the science of habit correction.

The very best book on that topic is *Atomic Habits*, and there is a reason it has spent 136 weeks on the *New York Times* Best Sellers List (and, of course, the number 136 is as of today—by the time you are reading this, the number will be higher).

A book doesn't spend 136+ weeks on the *New York Times* Best Sellers List unless it is remarkable.

I heard through the grapevine that James Clear is himself an intermittent faster, which didn't surprise me in the least, and when I looked into it, I learned he has actually written publicly about his intermittent fasting practice.

I can't do a better job writing about the science of habit creation than James Clear, so I won't even try. But because I am a teacher, I am going to summarize some of the points from his book that apply to your new intermittent fasting "habit":

- Your habits define you, whether you realize it or not. Everything you do over and over (often, without even thinking about it) is making your future *better* or *worse*. Think of some of your daily habits that you know are making your future better: you brush your teeth, you eat vegetables, you move your body. Just like those positive habits, intermittent fasting becomes a daily habit over time. As your intermittent fasting habit becomes second nature, and it will, it is most definitely making your future *better*.

19

- Habits shape your identity. To change your habits, focus on what you want to *become*. When you wake up every day and fast clean, open your eating window for a specified time, and then close it, it becomes who you are. It's more than what you *do*. It literally shapes your identity: you *are* an intermittent faster.
- Small changes add up. Even though you might not be able to see the changes that happen from day to day, they always show up in the long run, for better or for worse. Think about some of the chronic lifestyle diseases that have become so prevalent in our society. They are called *lifestyle diseases* because even though we may not want to hear it, they are based on decades of our choices, adding up. No one develops a chronic lifestyle disease overnight—it's based on long-term habits. When you live an intermittent fasting lifestyle, you're making small positive changes every day by fasting clean and delaying your eating window, and the positive effects on your body will definitely add up.
- Habits become automatic over time. James Clear says: "*The ultimate purpose of habits is to solve the problems*

of life with as little energy and effort as possible." To me, intermittent fasting is a perfect example of this concept. To be a successful intermittent faster, all you have to do is to *NOT* do something . . . don't eat, and then eat. Window closed, window open. Simple.

You may wonder how long it takes to build a new habit. I wish I could say, "It's twenty-eight days! Hooray!" Unfortunately, it isn't that simple. Pop culture tells us that it takes twenty-one days to form a new habit, but that number isn't based on science. It's just one of those "truths" that gets repeated enough times that everyone *believes* it's true.

What does the science actually say? A 2009 study called "How Are Habits Formed: Modeling Habit Formation in the Real World" found that the amount of time it takes to develop a habit that sticks can vary between 18 and 254 days. While that is hugely variable, the time required for the average person in the study was 66 days.

That study also found that you don't have to be perfect every single day for your habit to stick. That's good news for us, because it's hard to be "perfect," isn't it? I'm a firm believer that perfection is an illusion anyway.

We have a saying in our intermittent fasting community: Stop Stopping. As you keep living the intermittent fasting lifestyle for the next 66 to 254 days—however long it takes for it to become your habit—never forget that simple phrase. All you have to do is to *Keep Going*.

EXTRA CREDIT READING

Of course, the only extra credit reading you need is *Atomic Habits* by James Clear. Heck, with over ten million copies sold, you probably already have a copy somewhere around your house. Pull it out and read the first two chapters, and while you read, think about how what he is teaching you applies to your new intermittent fasting "habit." You can read more than the first two chapters, but the first two chapters will get you started.

DAILY INSPIRATION SPOTLIGHT:
Dennis Shock, Evans, Georgia
Intermittent Fasting Stories guest, episode 5

19

How long has he been an intermittent faster? *Over five years.*

Episode 5 of Intermittent Fasting Stories *was just after my one-year IF anniversary, also known as my fast-iversary. Gin and I spent time talking about where to go for burgers (because we share the love of a good burger!), and I explained what my IF journey looked like. I had started right in at fasting for over twenty hours per day and opened my eating window for only one to four hours per day from day 1. I rarely deviated from this. Perhaps once or twice a year for the first few years. November of 2022 marked five years of fasting for me. I still stick to this schedule during the week. My weekly window is usually only one to two hours a day. On the weekends, I generally eat two meals within three to five hours. I used to work from home, and now I go to the office every weekday. I don't find fasting to be harder in one scenario versus the other. My team at work knows I fast but cordially invite me to join in when they order out but expect me to say, "No, thank you." I lost about thirty pounds the first year (which was my goal) and to this day have kept off twenty-five of the thirty. I was an avid exerciser for the first few fasting years but have not made the time for that for the past two years. I still get on the scale every day—to keep myself honest. I have fasted for over thirty-five hours on two occasions but decided the long fasts are not for me. I try to keep my fasting times at twenty- to twenty-four-hour fasting periods. I work in the medical field in addition to being a self-published mystery suspense author. I'm fifty-eight years old, and I feel great. I'm in better physical shape than I was six years ago. I don't think I'll ever stop fasting. It's just part of who I am. I won't say it wasn't tough sometimes, starting out, but today, I do it with little thought to eating outside my window at all.*

ADVICE FROM DENNIS

Do your own research. You have to believe it's a healthy lifestyle like I do. Be open and honest about your fasting. Don't be afraid to talk about it. I believe it's a healthy way to live. You can make excuses, or you can be healthier. Research the barriers in your mind and find a way around them. Being active doesn't mean you can't fast. Feeling weak on a particular day doesn't mean you have to stop fasting forever. Consult your doctor. Tell the doctor you fast. They should be fully aware of what intermittent fasting is. I find it to be a great way of life.

**YOU HAVE ALL THE TOOLS YOU NEED TO SUCCEED.
ENJOY YOUR DAY! YOU'VE GOT THIS.**

HOW DID IT GO?
IT'S TIME TO REFLECT ON DAY 19.

TODAY (CHECK ALL THAT APPLY):

❏ I fasted clean (plain water, unflavored sparkling water, black unflavored coffee, plain tea)
❏ During the fast, I took time to reflect on the positive changes happening in my body
❏ Within my eating window, I ate until I was satisfied, and then I stopped
❏ I honored my "I've had enough" signals
❏ I stayed off the scale

FAST CHECK-IN

Rate the difficulty of today's fast on a scale from 1 to 10 (circle one):

1   2   3   4   5   6   7   8   9   **10**

(Today was easy! I sailed right through it.)   (Today was HARD! I struggled.)

During today's fast, I felt _____

_____

_____

_____

_____

_____

(*examples: exhilarated, hopeful, hungry, uncomfortable, bored, etc.*)

I used these strategies to manage my feelings today (check all that apply and add your own):

- ❏ I remembered my *why*
- ❏ I stayed busy
- ❏ I enjoyed a clean-fast-safe beverage
- ❏ I went on a walk
- ❏ I imagined my body tapping into my fat stores for fuel
- ❏ _____
  _____
- ❏ _____
  _____
- ❏ _____
  _____

EATING WINDOW CHECK-IN

Eating Window Length Goal: _____ hours
Actual Eating Window Length: _____ hours

How do I feel about today's eating window?

_____
_____
_____
_____
_____
_____
_____
_____
_____

What went well? Was there anything that I struggled with during my eating window? _____

_____

_____

_____

_____

_____

_____

_____

_____

_____

TODAY'S NSVS, OR NON-SCALE VICTORIES

One of the most powerful things we can do is acknowledge our Non-Scale Victories (NSVs). These can be physical (*pain reduction, better energy, mental clarity, etc.*) or emotional (*freedom around food, confidence, etc.*).

What were today's NSVs? _____

_____

_____

_____

_____

_____

_____

_____

_____

REFLECTIONS

Today, I listened to my body when I: _____

_____

_____

_____

_____

_____

_____

_____

Today's *AHA!* moment(s): _____

_____

_____

_____

Something that is on my mind: _____

_____

_____

_____

PREPARING FOR SUCCESS

Goal(s) and/or strategies for tomorrow: _____

_____

_____

_____

_____

DAY 20: YOU DIDN'T "FAIL"—WHEN THINGS DON'T GO ACCORDING TO PLAN

Today's Date: _____

PLANNING FOR A SUCCESSFUL DAY 20

20

Today, I am following

❏ The *Easy Does It* Approach (eight-hour window, including a low-carb ease-in lunch, plus a regular dinner)
❏ The *Steady Build* Approach (six-hour window, including lunch *or* snack, and dinner)
❏ The *Rip Off the Band-Aid* Approach (five-hour window, including lunch *or* snack, and dinner)

My personal goal(s) for today: _____
_____
_____
_____
_____
_____

Daily Lesson from Gin: You didn't "fail"—when things don't go according to plan.

No matter how great your intentions might be, there will always be times that things don't go according to plan. Maybe a planned eight-hour eating window stretches to twelve hours one day, or perhaps you intended to close your window with a healthy snack that turned into a carton of ice cream. Consider it to be a snaccident and move on.

Never compound one bad moment by giving in to thoughts such as "Well, I've ruined everything, so I might as well _____." You can fill in that blank with anything, such as "eat a whole pizza" or "finish the cookies."

We have all been there.

Instead of feeling like a failure and letting that feeling drive behaviors that make things even worse, take a deep breath and learn from it.

You know these familiar sayings: "Two wrongs don't make a right" and "Catch yourself before you wreck yourself." They apply here.

We learn more from mistakes than we learn from things that go according to plan.

Be teachable—and by that, I mean you're teaching *yourself* how your behaviors make you feel. Pay attention. How did you *feel* after that twelve-hour eating window or after that carton of ice cream? You probably didn't feel great, did you? Learn from that and keep going.

Feeling good is a powerful motivator, so keep doing things that make you *feel good*. And I am not talking about the transient and fake "feel good" moment you get while that carton of ice cream is going down. Once the carton is finished, you *don't* feel good, and I know you know what I mean. Maybe your stumbling block isn't ice cream, but we all have something that comes to mind.

Yesterday, you read about the science of habit creation, and I want to emphasize something that you learned.

In the research on habit creation, they found that it took 18–254 days for a habit to stick, but that doesn't mean that they had 18–254 "perfect" days in a row. Sticking to the new habit *most of the time* is what matters—a "bad day" didn't force the clock to start over.

Now, take that same lesson and apply it to your 28-Day FAST Start.

If you have a bad day (or even a string of less-than-successful days) you didn't fail, and even more important: you aren't starting over.

In fact, let's make a pact: I would like for you to *never again* use the words *starting over* when it comes to your intermittent fasting lifestyle.

The 28-Day FAST Start isn't something you should plan to do over and over—it's something to use to get started, and it's a time for your body to learn to flip the metabolic switch.

I'm not such a wide-eyed optimist that I think no one will *ever* stop fasting and restart, of course. But the goal of going through the FAST Start (and this book, in particular) is to make sure that your intermittent fasting lifestyle *sticks*.

Your mindset is a HUGE part of that (more about mindset on day 23).

So, what do you do when something doesn't go according to plan? Here's an example: maybe you make it to day 26 of your FAST Start and then you have a five-day hiccup and go back to eating all day long for those days.

What should you do?

Keep going.

You always just keep going.

In that example, if you had twenty-six successful days in a row, pick right back up with day 27, even with that hiccup in between.

The worst thing that might happen is that you have

delayed the amount of time it takes for your body to become fat adapted.

You're not running a race here—you are building a new habit. Whether it takes you 18, 66, or 254 days to get it right, the most important thing you can do is remember this:

No matter what happened today, tomorrow you'll wake up in the fasted state and have a fresh new clean fast.

Simply keep going.

EXTRA CREDIT READING

Chapter 19 of *Fast. Feast. Repeat.*, which is called "Lifestyle Versus Diet: There Is No Wagon." When you stumble, you didn't "fall off the wagon." We can't "fall off" a lifestyle, am I right?

DAILY INSPIRATION SPOTLIGHT:
Melody Patrick, Harrisburg, Pennsylvania
Intermittent Fasting Stories guest, episode 27

How long has she been an intermittent faster? *Over five years.*

It was 2016 when I stumbled upon intermittent fasting while searching for ways to simplify my life and help rein in my tendency to eat from a place of boredom or anxiety. However, I quickly became intrigued as the world of IF opened up to me—reduced inflammation and infection, a strengthened immune system, and this thing called autophagy! As someone who has suffered with Crohn's disease since being diagnosed in 1986, at the age of twenty, this was revolutionary to me! And so my IF journey began. The more I studied the healing potential of fasting, the more it made sense to me. I was familiar with fasting as a spiritual discipline. If fasting is good for the spirit, why would it not also benefit my entire well-being? I was all in! Initially, I began fasting for eighteen hours a day, but soon moved to twenty. I not only saved time and money, I experienced improvements in my overall wellness—even through seasons of anxiety, unemployment, a death in the family, and health challenges my husband was facing. Through it all, intermittent fasting was one of the tools God gave to guide me. Today, as a woman in her late fifties, I continue to practice a twenty- to twenty-one-hour daily fast, with some flexibility on weekends and vacations and a monthly forty-eight-hour fast. I focus on eating clean (most of the time), prayer, and cultivating strong relationships. I have managed my Crohn's disease without medication since 2013. I also thank God for Gin and others like her, who are getting the word out to people such as myself, that we may experience a healthier, more abundant life!

ADVICE FROM MELODY

Be encouraged, because it's never too late to start making better choices! God has given you your mind, body, talents, friends, environment—even your challenges—as a gift. No matter what is in your past, what mistakes or failures you have made or experienced, His mercy is new each morning—in fasting, in relationships, in life!

**YOU HAVE ALL THE TOOLS YOU NEED TO SUCCEED.
ENJOY YOUR DAY! YOU'VE GOT THIS.**

HOW DID IT GO?
IT'S TIME TO REFLECT ON DAY 20.

TODAY (CHECK ALL THAT APPLY):

❏ I fasted clean (plain water, unflavored sparkling water, black unflavored coffee, plain tea)
❏ During the fast, I took time to reflect on the positive changes happening in my body
❏ Within my eating window, I ate until I was satisfied, and then I stopped
❏ I honored my "I've had enough" signals
❏ I stayed off the scale

FAST CHECK-IN

Rate the difficulty of today's fast on a scale from 1 to 10 (circle one):

1 2 3 4 5 6 7 8 9 **10**

(Today was easy! I sailed right through it.)   (Today was HARD! I struggled.)

During today's fast, I felt _____

_____

_____

_____

_____

_____

(*examples: exhilarated, hopeful, hungry, uncomfortable, bored, etc.*)

I used these strategies to manage my feelings today (check all that apply and add your own):

❏ I remembered my *why*
❏ I stayed busy
❏ I enjoyed a clean-fast-safe beverage
❏ I went on a walk
❏ I imagined my body tapping into my fat stores for fuel
❏ _____

_____
❏ _____

_____
❏ _____

_____

EATING WINDOW CHECK-IN

Eating Window Length Goal: _____ hours
Actual Eating Window Length: _____ hours

How do I feel about today's eating window?

_____
_____
_____
_____
_____
_____
_____
_____
_____
_____

What went well? Was there anything that I struggled with during my eating window? _____

_____

_____

_____

_____

_____

_____

_____

_____

_____

TODAY'S NSVS, OR NON-SCALE VICTORIES

One of the most powerful things we can do is acknowledge our Non-Scale Victories (NSVs). These can be physical (*pain reduction, better energy, mental clarity, etc.*) or emotional (*freedom around food, confidence, etc.*).

What were today's NSVs? _____

_____

_____

_____

_____

_____

_____

_____

_____

REFLECTIONS

Today, I listened to my body when I: _____

_____

_____

_____

_____

_____

_____

_____

_____

Today's *AHA!* moment(s): _____

_____

_____

_____

Something that is on my mind: _____

_____

_____

_____

PREPARING FOR SUCCESS

Goal(s) and/or strategies for tomorrow: _____

_____

_____

_____

_____

_____

DAY 21: NEGATIVE NELLIES (AND WHY WE *SHARE WITHOUT FEAR* ANYWAY)

Today's Date: _____

PLANNING FOR A SUCCESSFUL DAY 21

Today, I am following

- ❏ The *Easy Does It* Approach (eight-hour window, including a low-carb ease-in lunch, plus a regular dinner)
- ❏ The *Steady Build* Approach (six-hour window, including lunch *or* snack, and dinner)
- ❏ The *Rip Off the Band-Aid* Approach (five-hour window, including lunch *or* snack, and dinner)

My personal goal(s) for today: _____

_____

_____

_____

_____

Daily Lesson from Gin: Negative Nellies (and why we *share without fear* anyway).

First of all, if your name is Nellie, I want to apologize to you up front. I am sure *you* are delightful and not at all negative. I'm talking about all of those other "negative Nellies" out there, who aren't even actually named Nellie. Being a "negative Nellie" is a mindset problem.

As you get deeper into your intermittent fasting lifestyle, you'll probably start feeling so good that you'll want to shout it from the rooftops. Not only is fasting free, but when you live an IF lifestyle, you're empowered to take charge of your own health. You learn what makes you feel great and what foods work best for your body, and you finally begin to lose the diet-brain chatter that may have been with you for years or even decades. Nagging health conditions start to clear up, and you lose weight. You've never felt better.

So, imagine this scenario. You are hanging out with a good friend or family member who notices you look and feel great (thanks to the IF glow that follows you everywhere), and then they mention they are dieting or struggling with a health issue, and you feel like it's a great time to tell them about intermittent fasting . . . only to receive a lot of pushback, including phrases like "You're starving yourself," "That isn't healthy," or "Everyone knows breakfast is the most important meal of the day."

Sigh. Negative Nellie has arrived.

Maybe they start scouring the internet for videos or blog posts that "prove" that IF is "dangerous," and they send them to you whenever they can find them.

We've actually experienced a recent flurry of that last scenario. In the fall of 2022, a study came out that led to sensationalistic headlines that implied fasting makes you more likely to die.

In our IF community, concerned fasters started sharing the articles. Was fasting going to make them DIE? That didn't sound like what they signed up for.

So, of course, we looked at the study.

When you look at any study, one of the most important

things to do is to look at who funded or published it. This particular study was published by the Academy of Nutrition and Dietetics. Who are they? According to their website, some of their donors include companies such as the American Egg Board, the Kellogg Company, and General Mills, among others you would probably recognize.

Ah. So, an organization supported by Big Food companies (who have a vested interest in you eating breakfast) published a study that tells us we shouldn't fast. That's interesting.

Still, the headlines were alarming. I don't want to be more likely to die.

Logically, that doesn't make a lot of sense. Was I "more likely to die" when I weighed 210 pounds and was obese, or am I "more likely to die" now that I am at a healthy weight, with excellent health biomarkers? We all know the answer to that.

After learning who published the study and moving past the headlines, it was time to dig deeper into the methodology. It turns out, they relied on asking people how they ate and then linked their responses to health outcomes.

The people who said they skipped meals did tend to have poor overall health outcomes. But let's dig in a bit more.

The people who self-reported as "skipping meals" tended to be drinkers and smokers, and they also reported food insecurity. This makes it likely that they were not receiving adequate nutrition when they did eat. It's really hard to know, especially when you're basing conclusions on self-reported data. People are not great at self-reporting over time.

Another important point to keep in mind is that skipping meals is not the same thing as fasting. Not even close. One example of this is a friend of mine who recently told me she "does that fasting thing" that I do and she only eats dinner. But when we talked about it in greater detail, she told me she drinks a green juice first thing in the morning, puts cream in her coffee, and drinks fruit- and lemon-infused water all day. Is she fasting? Nope. Does she think she is fasting? Yes, she does.

Had my friend been interviewed for that study, she would have said she only eats one meal a day. Actually, she is on an extremely low-calorie diet all day long (green juice, creamy coffee, and fruity water), and then she's having one meal of solid food. The beverages keep her insulin levels high, and you probably recall me mentioning the excellent book *Why We Get Sick* that explains the link between chronically high levels of insulin and all sorts of modern diseases.

To lower insulin levels, we need to do a lot more than "skip meals." We need to *fast clean*. The two are not at all the same thing.

This study leaves us with a lot of questions about the participants, but what it doesn't do is tell us anything about fasting, even though the headlines screamed otherwise.

The moral of this story is that you can't take headlines at face value these days. Those articles with sensational headlines like "Intermittent Fasting Will Make You Die" got a lot of clicks and shares, whereas an article with a more realistic title such as "People Who Don't Eat Nutritious Foods Because of Food Insecurity and Other Poor

Lifestyle Habits Are More Likely to Die" wouldn't feel like much of a story. (Though, as a side note, it actually is a *very big* story. If we could improve the nutrition of the world and eliminate the overwhelming reliance on ultra-processed foods, it would change the entire health landscape for the better. It's not in anyone's financial interests to tell you that story. "Eat more real food" is boring and doesn't inspire very many clicks.)

The reason I mentioned this study from 2022 is that there will always be confusing news stories or negative Nellies who want to convince you that you really need to eat all day long, and in the case of Big Food, they particularly want to convince you that you need to eat (or drink) whatever they are selling.

Instead of letting this type of thing confuse or upset you, I want you to be confident that IF is a healthy way to live. For me, nothing has been more of a confirmation of the power of IF than the way I feel. I feel too amazing, and I'm too healthy for this to be "bad" for me.

Listen to your body. If you feel better than you've felt in a long time, that's a good sign. Ignore the negative Nellies, and trust in your body's wisdom.

And always share without fear . . . even though you might run across a negative Nellie. Vow that you aren't going to let them get inside your head if and when that happens. But instead of getting pushback, you might just change someone's life. There is no better feeling than that.

DAILY INSPIRATION SPOTLIGHT:
Deb Crosby, Ottawa, Ontario, Canada
Intermittent Fasting Stories guest, episode 208

21

How long has she been an intermittent faster? *Between two and three years.*

My journey toward intermittent fasting started after my first pregnancy. I had always been a curvy teen, but very active. As a teen, I noticed I always felt better if I didn't eat breakfast (this comes into play later). I have had three pregnancies, and the weight gained with each pregnancy became increasingly harder to take off. Up until August of 2020, I am sure I had tried ALL the different diets! I even tried medication to try to take the weight off. I would lose weight, but as soon as I stopped following the plan, I would gain the weight back plus more. Prior to IF, I would become hangry and shaky if I didn't eat every few hours. My daughter even gave my wife a tip when she first met her. She said always have snacks for Mom! (Insert eye roll here! LOL.) The year 2020 was very difficult for everyone, due to the pandemic and being isolated at home. In my case, my spouse was deployed to the Middle East. I also sustained a knee injury and was unable to work at my active nursing job, so I was sad, lonely, and eating a lot. Right before my wife returned, I was at my highest weight ever, and I was horrified! One day, I had to crawl out of the tub and thought, This cannot be my life. I decided something had to give, so I googled how to lose weight (yet again), and I found Gin's first book, Delay, Don't Deny. I devoured it and knew this was for me! I immediately started at 16:8 and found it to be quite simple. The hardest thing to do was to give up the cream in my coffee. The bonus was I was no longer HANGRY! I continued fasting and quickly discovered that I needed to weigh every day rather than once a week, and I watched that trend go down slowly. If I looked at the weight trend on an app, it was like a sawtooth with up days and down days. Focusing on the trend made all the difference. My wife joined me in this journey in December of 2020. In February of 2022, I was so excited to be on Gin's Intermittent Fasting Stories *podcast, episode 208. It was so much fun! We discussed my journey and me being a "turtle," meaning very slow to lose the weight. This is key: so many people want a quick fix, but there isn't one. Just look at long-range success. My starting weight was 236 pounds, and I'm five foot three. I'm writing this in January of 2023, I'm back working in a busy ER, and I have lost 50 pounds. I've gone through three Christmases now and not gained that weight back! It's just so simple, I feel like I have the tools to understand what I need to do to ensure that weight does not return.*

ADVICE FROM DEB

For new fasters just starting, I suggest you don't get hung up on the weight. Just drink lots of plain or sparkling water, fast every day clean, meaning no cream in your coffee (yes, you can do it), and listen to your body. I found if I had a carb-heavy meal one day, the next day I was hungrier than if I had eaten a nutrient-dense meal. Stop when you are full. Even if there is food left. If you find a day where you ate more than you wanted to, don't be discouraged, because the next day is a new day. There is no "wagon to fall off of." There ARE planned indulgences, so eat that birthday cake with NO guilt! It is a way of life and a way of eating, and you just get started again the next day. You CAN do it!

21

**YOU HAVE ALL THE TOOLS YOU NEED TO SUCCEED.
ENJOY YOUR DAY! YOU'VE GOT THIS.**

HOW DID IT GO?
IT'S TIME TO REFLECT ON DAY 21.

TODAY (CHECK ALL THAT APPLY):

❏ I fasted clean (plain water, unflavored sparkling water, black unflavored coffee, plain tea)
❏ During the fast, I took time to reflect on the positive changes happening in my body
❏ Within my eating window, I ate until I was satisfied, and then I stopped
❏ I honored my "I've had enough" signals
❏ I stayed off the scale

FAST CHECK-IN

Rate the difficulty of today's fast on a scale from 1 to 10 (circle one):

1　2　3　4　5　6　7　8　9　**10**

(Today was easy! I sailed right through it.)　　(Today was HARD! I struggled.)

During today's fast, I felt _____

_____

_____

_____

_____

_____

(*examples: exhilarated, hopeful, hungry, uncomfortable, bored, etc.*)

I used these strategies to manage my feelings today (check all that apply and add your own):

- ❏ I remembered my *why*
- ❏ I stayed busy
- ❏ I enjoyed a clean-fast-safe beverage
- ❏ I went on a walk
- ❏ I imagined my body tapping into my fat stores for fuel
- ❏ _____
  _____
- ❏ _____
  _____
- ❏ _____
  _____

EATING WINDOW CHECK-IN

Eating Window Length Goal: _____ hours
Actual Eating Window Length: _____ hours

How do I feel about today's eating window?

_____
_____
_____
_____
_____
_____
_____
_____
_____
_____

What went well? Was there anything that I struggled with during my eating window? _____

_____

_____

_____

_____

_____

_____

_____

_____

_____

TODAY'S NSVS, OR NON-SCALE VICTORIES

One of the most powerful things we can do is acknowledge our Non-Scale Victories (NSVs). These can be physical (*pain reduction, better energy, mental clarity, etc.*) or emotional (*freedom around food, confidence, etc.*).

What were today's NSVs? _____

_____

_____

_____

_____

_____

_____

_____

_____

REFLECTIONS

Today, I listened to my body when I: _____

_____

_____

_____

_____

_____

_____

_____

Today's *AHA!* moment(s): _____

_____

_____

_____

_____

Something that is on my mind: _____

_____

_____

_____

_____

PREPARING FOR SUCCESS

Goal(s) and/or strategies for tomorrow: _____

_____

_____

_____

_____

_____

WEEK 4 PLAN

Which approach did you choose for last week?

☐ The *Easy Does It* Approach (eight-hour window, including a low-carb ease-in lunch, plus a regular dinner)

☐ The *Steady Build* Approach (six-hour window, including lunch *or* snack, and dinner)

☐ The *Rip Off the Band-Aid* Approach (five-hour window, including lunch *or* snack, and dinner)

How did it go?

☐ It was too easy! I think I can ramp it up this week.

☐ It was JUST RIGHT. Not too hard, not too easy.

☐ It was too much for me. I am going to scale it back this week.

Which approach will you follow for week 4?

☐ The *Easy Does It* Approach (six-hour window, including a low-carb ease-in lunch *or* snack, plus a regular dinner)

☐ The *Steady Build* Approach (five-hour window, including snack, and dinner)

☐ The *Rip Off the Band-Aid* Approach (four-hour window, including snack, and dinner)

Thirty

DAY 22: ARE WE THERE YET? FLIPPING YOUR METABOLIC SWITCH

Today's Date: _____

PLANNING FOR A SUCCESSFUL DAY 22

Today, I am following

❏ The *Easy Does It* Approach (six-hour window, including a low-carb ease-in lunch *or* snack, plus a regular dinner)
❏ The *Steady Build* Approach (five-hour window, including snack, and dinner)
❏ The *Rip Off the Band-Aid* Approach (four-hour window, including snack, and dinner)

My personal goal(s) for today: _____

_____

_____

_____

_____

Daily Lesson from Gin: Are we there yet? Flipping your metabolic switch.

On day 9, I explained the process of flipping your metabolic switch, and I want to revisit that topic today. It's been almost two weeks since I explained the process, and you may be wondering if you're there yet. It's likely that you are *not,* which probably makes you wonder when it will finally happen.

In fact, you may be reaching the point of the FAST Start where fasting actually gets harder before it gets easier again. Maybe that already happened, maybe it's happening today, or maybe it is still in your future. No matter which is true for you, it really helps to understand what is happening.

Remember that when the metabolic switch is flipped, our bodies go from running on glucose (from the foods we eat and our stored glycogen) to running on the fat from our fat stores and also the ketones that are produced to fuel our brains.

The big question is this: At what point do our bodies flip this metabolic switch? It happens when our liver glycogen has been sufficiently depleted and fat cells are mobilized to meet our energy needs.

Remember the visual I gave you on day 9: think of the liver as a glycogen storage tank. When we eat, we use food for fuel and store the extra away for later. Some of this excess goes into our liver and muscles as stored glycogen, while some may be stored away as fat. When we fast, we switch over to using our backup fuel sources for energy, and when we don't have enough glycogen left to fuel us, our bodies have no choice but to dip into stored fat. Voilà! Metabolic flexibility, just as nature intended!

It's now day 22, and you may be wondering when your body will make this transition. Unfortunately, as I already mentioned, it varies greatly from person to person. The 28-Day FAST Start is designed so that most new IFers will flip that metabolic switch by day 28, but it can be sooner (or longer) than twenty-eight days for some bodies. If you have been metabolically unhealthy for a while, it will likely take you longer to adapt than a body that is already somewhat metabolically healthy.

As I already explained, as you continue to go along from day to day, you will usually reach a point where fasting gets harder again before it gets easier. This is normal. It's actually a good sign when that happens, because it indicates your body is just about to flip the metabolic switch.

If it already happened: celebrate! The physically hard part is behind you. If it hasn't happened yet, hang in there. It may take longer than twenty-eight days for your body to flip the metabolic switch, but you'll get there at your body's pace.

DAILY INSPIRATION SPOTLIGHT:
Anne-Lise Jasinski, Joplin, Missouri
Intermittent Fasting Stories guest, episode 139

How long has she been an intermittent faster? *Over five years.*

I grew up with a very troubled relationship with food. There was a lot of shame and pressure around weight and body image in my family of origin. Additionally, fasting was part of our religious practice. When I became an adult, I abandoned that religion and as many of the pressures about my body as I could. After being abandoned by an abusive husband at thirty years old, I met and married my soulmate, experiencing unconditional love for the first time. I promptly gained sixty pounds. I found IF in 2017 and went all in. It was the first time I had experienced an actual break from my relationship with food. While fasting, I was able to stop the madness of food obsession by just NOT eating at all. That time of rest between eating windows has proven to be absolutely life-changing. While my first few years of IF were coupled with extended water fasts and a strict keto protocol, I have since relaxed my approach. I switched to OMAD for several years, enjoying the simplicity of such a short eating window, which, again, gave me large breaks from the decision fatigue associated with food choices. In the past year or so, I have been healing the last layers of residual diet culture trauma. I now have a loose 18:6 window with no food restrictions. I enjoy naturally breaking my fast when I get hungry, usually between noon and 3:00 p.m. I prefer a well-balanced meal with high-quality, nutrient-dense food. I enjoy a "mini-fast" until my evening meal, which is less structured. I love to be done eating by 7:00 or 8:00 p.m., which helps me sleep more soundly and avoid a morning food hangover. My relationship with food is still healing, and IF is an ongoing tool in that process. I am forever grateful to Gin and her dedication to education for bringing so much supportive information and encouragement to the world.

ADVICE FROM ANNE-LISE

IF is as natural as eating. Consider looking at it as a healthy and integral part of your relationship with food. Enjoying a fasting window creates an ideal contrast that allows you to fall in love with eating again. Food becomes a more conscious choice. The act of eating can then become an intentional expression of self-love that helps you inhabit and heal your body at ever-deepening levels. Fast on!

**YOU HAVE ALL THE TOOLS YOU NEED TO SUCCEED.
ENJOY YOUR DAY! YOU'VE GOT THIS.**

HOW DID IT GO?
IT'S TIME TO REFLECT ON DAY 22.

TODAY (CHECK ALL THAT APPLY):

- ❏ I fasted clean (plain water, unflavored sparkling water, black unflavored coffee, plain tea)
- ❏ During the fast, I took time to reflect on the positive changes happening in my body
- ❏ Within my eating window, I ate until I was satisfied, and then I stopped
- ❏ I honored my "I've had enough" signals
- ❏ I stayed off the scale

FAST CHECK-IN

Rate the difficulty of today's fast on a scale from 1 to 10 (circle one):

1 2 3 4 5 6 7 8 9 **10**

(Today was easy! I sailed right through it.)   (Today was HARD! I struggled.)

During today's fast, I felt _____

_____

_____

_____

_____

(*examples: exhilarated, hopeful, hungry, uncomfortable, bored, etc.*)

I used these strategies to manage my feelings today (check all that apply and add your own):

- ❏ I remembered my *why*
- ❏ I stayed busy
- ❏ I enjoyed a clean-fast-safe beverage
- ❏ I went on a walk
- ❏ I imagined my body tapping into my fat stores for fuel
- ❏ _____
  _____
- ❏ _____
  _____
- ❏ _____
  _____

EATING WINDOW CHECK-IN

Eating Window Length Goal: _____ hours
Actual Eating Window Length: _____ hours

How do I feel about today's eating window?

_____
_____
_____
_____
_____
_____
_____
_____
_____
_____

What went well? Was there anything that I struggled with during my eating window? _____

_____

_____

_____

_____

_____

_____

_____

_____

_____

TODAY'S NSVS, OR NON-SCALE VICTORIES

One of the most powerful things we can do is acknowledge our Non-Scale Victories (NSVs). These can be physical (*pain reduction, better energy, mental clarity, etc.*) or emotional (*freedom around food, confidence, etc.*).

What were today's NSVs? _____

_____

_____

_____

_____

_____

_____

_____

_____

REFLECTIONS

Today, I listened to my body when I: _____

_____

_____

_____

_____

_____

_____

_____

Today's *AHA!* moment(s): _____

_____

_____

_____

_____

Something that is on my mind: _____

_____

_____

_____

_____

PREPARING FOR SUCCESS

Goal(s) and/or strategies for tomorrow: _____

_____

_____

_____

_____

_____

DAY 23: FOCUSING ON MINDSET FOR THE LONG HAUL

Today's Date: _____

PLANNING FOR A SUCCESSFUL DAY 23

Today, I am following

- ❏ The *Easy Does It* Approach (six-hour window, including a low-carb ease-in lunch *or* snack, plus a regular dinner)
- ❏ The *Steady Build* Approach (five-hour window, including snack, and dinner)
- ❏ The *Rip Off the Band-Aid* Approach (four-hour window, including snack, and dinner)

My personal goal(s) for today: _____

_____

_____

_____

_____

Daily Lesson from Gin: Focusing on mindset for the long haul

Whether you think you can or you think you can't, you're right.

I am sure you've heard that saying before, and it's attributed to Henry Ford. It's a powerful quote because it's true, and science backs this idea up.

The book that first opened my eyes to the importance of

our inner dialogue is *Mindset* by Carol Dweck. Dr. Dweck is a psychologist whose life's work is focused on the areas of motivation, personality, and social development.

She describes two distinct mindsets: the fixed mindset and the growth mindset.

When someone has a fixed mindset, they believe that they have specific abilities or traits that are set, and therefore out of their control.

A growth mindset, on the other hand, reflects a belief that through hard work and perseverance, you can change. You have a great deal of control when it comes to your future.

Dr. Dweck's initial work relates to the concept of intelligence, abilities, and talents and can absolutely be applied to our intermittent fasting lifestyles.

Which of these two thoughts is most like what you tell yourself?

Example 1: *Weight loss is a struggle for me. Intermittent fasting probably won't work, just as nothing else I've ever tried has worked. I'm destined to be overweight forever.*

OR

Example 2: *I may have struggled in the past, but I believe that intermittent fasting is changing my destiny. I know that my body can become metabolically flexible, and I have the tools to tweak it till it's easy and work with my body to reach a healthy weight forever.*

I'm sure you can figure out that the first would be an example of a fixed mindset, whereas the other is an example of a growth mindset, as applied to intermittent fasting.

I've been managing online peer-to-peer intermittent fasting support communities since 2015, and I can tell you that mindset matters. Strugglers struggle, and overcomers overcome.

The words you tell yourself matter.

Your beliefs. They *matter.*

Right now, today, I want you to craft a belief statement about your future as an intermittent faster.

23

If you are like example 1 from above, and you currently have a struggle-focused fixed mindset, push yourself out of your comfort zone and force yourself to write a growth-mindset-oriented belief statement. Even if it feels like a total lie, write it down anyway. You can copy example 2 word for word if you need to. Or you can make it completely your own.

My belief statement:

_____

_____

_____

_____

EXTRA CREDIT READING

Chapter 20 of *Fast. Feast. Repeat.* is an in-depth look at the power of mindset. In that chapter, I share even more of the science that supports the importance of your thoughts. Success really does come from within, but so does failure. Begin thinking like a success story, and you'll change your life forever.

DAILY INSPIRATION SPOTLIGHT:
Piper Brinkley, Mauldin, South Carolina
Intermittent Fasting Stories guest, episode 51

How long has she been an intermittent faster? *Over five years.*

Shortly after my episode aired in October 2019, I wound up initiating a divorce for a major life change. Thanks to the clarity of being alcohol-free, I was able to see my marriage for what it was and decided that it was in the best interest of my son and I to separate from my spouse. Then, of course, in 2020, the pandemic hit! As everyone knows, this brought the world to a standstill. I leaned heavily on my fasting and alcohol-free lifestyle (IF+AF) at this point to get me through. During this worldwide challenge, my daily fasts and clear mind were just the structure and discipline I required to keep my sanity. And some days, that was about all I had! Even with the stress of the ongoing divorce while running our shared company with my "wasband" during a pandemic with a young child, my homelife was much improved. I was able to publish my book on Amazon, Tips, Tricks, & Tweaks for the IF Lifestyle, *which was a proud moment for me. The purpose is to help people to join forces with their bodies and become allies with their bodies. Fasting is a powerful way to do just that! I connected with my Intermittent Fasting & Alcohol-Free Lifestyle Facebook group daily for support. The group is filled with supportive people that let go of alcohol and find that doing so just supercharges their fasting and their lives! The personal growth and self-love that blossom out of this process are so rewarding to witness. With my little family being just my son and myself, I was finally able to feel peaceful and calm in my home. What a contrast and relief! It is interesting once this feeling of safety was established, my body actually let some weight/size go. This taught me the critical impact of stress on my body and the importance of minimizing excess stress and how important it is to shed all toxic things from my life. Stress relief/management then became my focus. I did all the basic things to minimize the stress that was occurring in my life and the world. I learned and added so many coping skills and*

23

reached out for help when I needed it. These past several years have been the hardest yet the most rewarding and the most intense period of growth as well. I could not have done it without my clear head and healthy lifestyle. IF+AF has been the foundation of this incredible healing journey that my body has benefited from as well. My body guided me all along my fasting journey to establish the protocols necessary for any given period of my life. My body also guided me to let go of alcohol, as it added nothing of value to my life and wasn't tolerated well at all. And anything else toxic that no longer serves me as well! The IF+AF lifestyle has catapulted me into a new relationship with myself. This has been so empowering! My body then showed me that stress could impact my body's functioning drastically. I have learned that when my body is less stressed, everything else is just easier and my body is happier. When it is happy, I look and feel great! Really focusing on exercise, sleep, and being present has done so much to complement IF+AF to bring me toward my healthiest, most vibrant self. Every single thing in my life has improved with this lifestyle. I have been in maintenance for a very long time, and yet my body still adjusts to what it requires. My protocol has been refined throughout these last four years, depending on what my body calls for or requires. Life is happening all the time, and our bodies adapt—thank goodness! I have continued to shed sizes. I am more of a size 2–4 and fit into what I wore in college and weigh the same as well, in the low 120s. (This is down six to ten pounds from my previous maintenance weight, so my body is still changing since 2014.) I have noticed that the closer I get to my authentic self, the more my body adjusts to the most efficient shape and size. Although I do not own a scale, I see my weight at the doctor's office. I take the scale reading in with curiosity and compare it to how I feel in my clothes and in my life. It usually corresponds, and that's about it. The scale does not dictate my success in this lifestyle, but my body's feelings of satiety, peace, and vibrancy do! That's what I focus on—the feels! I continue to be amazed at the flexibility of this lifestyle and the simplicity and joy it brings to all my days. Throughout my journey, my size/weight has changed. Life is not stagnant, and neither is my body. I have adjusted my protocols accordingly to keep where my body feels happiest. Sometimes, stretching my window to 16:8 to ease the stressful impact on my body, and sometimes having longer (thirty-six- to forty-two-hour) fasts, one to two times per week. Now, I am primarily a daily-window gal, with one- to four-hour daily windows. I move for joy daily. I have gotten very in tune to what my body requires daily (loads of greens, delicious protein, starch/legumes) at a minimum. So, my plate is pretty formulaic, and my windows are much more efficient but no less scrumptious. I still open with my plated meal and have a snack and/or dessert a bit later. Some days are earlier and some later; some windows are shorter and some longer. That's all there is to it!

ADVICE FROM PIPER

If you are starting back or even just struggling on your IF journey, take a moment and realize that you can't do everything in one fast or one eating window. So, take it one fast at a time. One window at a time! That's it. One day at a time and one step at a time! Consistency doesn't mean identical daily. It just means you fast every day. The best thing about IF is the freedom from the diet mentality, so let go of the restrictions that *cause you stress and angst. There are no mistakes or messing up. Keep the fast clean; that's it. Listen to your body because your body is your guide. Eat what makes your body feel great. Super simple. And . . . it is easy to start; you can begin again just as soon as you stop eating!*

23

YOU HAVE ALL THE TOOLS YOU NEED TO SUCCEED. ENJOY YOUR DAY! YOU'VE GOT THIS.

HOW DID IT GO?
IT'S TIME TO REFLECT ON DAY 23.

TODAY (CHECK ALL THAT APPLY):

❏ I fasted clean (plain water, unflavored sparkling water, black unflavored coffee, plain tea)
❏ During the fast, I took time to reflect on the positive changes happening in my body
❏ Within my eating window, I ate until I was satisfied, and then I stopped
❏ I honored my "I've had enough" signals
❏ I stayed off the scale

FAST CHECK-IN

Rate the difficulty of today's fast on a scale from 1 to 10 (circle one):

1   2   3   4   5   6   7   8   9   **10**

(Today was easy! I sailed right through it.)   (Today was HARD! I struggled.)

During today's fast, I felt _____

_____

_____

_____

_____

(*examples: exhilarated, hopeful, hungry, uncomfortable, bored, etc.*)

I used these strategies to manage my feelings today (check all that apply and add your own):

- ❏ I remembered my *why*
- ❏ I stayed busy
- ❏ I enjoyed a clean-fast-safe beverage
- ❏ I went on a walk
- ❏ I imagined my body tapping into my fat stores for fuel
- ❏ _____
  _____
- ❏ _____
  _____
- ❏ _____
  _____

EATING WINDOW CHECK-IN

Eating Window Length Goal: _____ hours
Actual Eating Window Length: _____ hours

How do I feel about today's eating window?

_____
_____
_____
_____
_____
_____
_____
_____
_____
_____

What went well? Was there anything that I struggled with during my eating window? _____

_____

_____

_____

_____

_____

_____

_____

_____

TODAY'S NSVS, OR NON-SCALE VICTORIES

One of the most powerful things we can do is acknowledge our Non-Scale Victories (NSVs). These can be physical (*pain reduction, better energy, mental clarity, etc.*) or emotional (*freedom around food, confidence, etc.*).

What were today's NSVs? _____

_____

_____

_____

_____

_____

_____

_____

_____

REFLECTIONS

Today, I listened to my body when I: _____

_____

_____

_____

_____

_____

_____

_____

Today's *AHA!* moment(s): _____

_____

_____

_____

Something that is on my mind: _____

_____

_____

_____

PREPARING FOR SUCCESS

Goal(s) and/or strategies for tomorrow: _____

_____

_____

_____

_____

DAY 24: THE IMPORTANCE OF REALISTIC EXPECTATIONS

Today's Date: _____

PLANNING FOR A SUCCESSFUL DAY 24

Today, I am following

- ❏ The *Easy Does It* Approach (six-hour window, including a low-carb ease-in lunch *or* snack, plus a regular dinner)
- ❏ The *Steady Build* Approach (five-hour window, including snack, and dinner)
- ❏ The *Rip Off the Band-Aid* Approach (four-hour window, including snack, and dinner)

My personal goal(s) for today: _____

_____

_____

_____

_____

Daily Lesson from Gin: The importance of realistic expectations

I've already told you this important truth: the 28-Day FAST Start is *not* the time to expect weight loss. Because of this, I encourage you not to weigh during the FAST Start. You committed to that promise before you began, and I hope you have followed through.

But here we are on day 24, and I bet you're secretly thinking about what you'll see when you get on the scale on day 29. You're probably hoping to see a big drop in that number. I get it. I would hope for that, too.

And that is why today's lesson is on realistic expectations.

Just for fun (although it actually makes me more than a little mad, and that doesn't feel very fun), I searched for some headlines from the types of magazines you see at the supermarket checkout. I am not making these up: these are the real headlines (though I cut them down just a bit for brevity without changing any of their words or claims).

24

- No-Work Weight Loss: Feel Better Than Ever as You Lose 23 Lbs. in 14 Days
- Super-Nutrient "Unlocks" Fat Cells to Speed-Shrink Your Midsection: Lose 25 Pounds in 10 Days
- Boost Metabolism by 1,000%! Lose 32 Lbs. in 2 Weeks!
- Doctor's Best Diet Soup: Lose 24 Lbs. This Week!
- Better Than Gastric Bypass: You Could Reverse Type 2 Diabetes and Drop 60 Lbs. in 30 Days

I could go on and on, because we have all seen these magazines. I used to buy them, just like you may have. I would flip right to the article featured on the cover, and there was usually a diet book or product I needed to buy.

I was *so ready* to lose twenty-three pounds in fourteen days, or even better, twenty-four pounds this week! Sixty pounds in thirty days? Yes, please!

The headlines claimed it was possible, so why couldn't it happen for me?

Here's why: it is impossible to lose fat that quickly. It literally can't happen.

Weight loss and *fat loss* are two different things, of course, though most people don't think about that distinction. We are so used to getting on the scale and taking that number at face value. If it is up, we must have gained fat. If it's down, we assume we have lost fat.

The number on the scale is about so much more than how much fat is on your body. It's the sum of all your fat tissue, lean tissue, the amount of water within your body, your organs, food in your digestive system, and so on. Any quick upward or downward swings are not a reflection of fat gain or loss, because we gain or lose fat very slowly.

How quickly *can* we lose fat? That is a great question. The value varies from person to person and depends on individual factors, such as metabolic rate, what you're eating, your daily energy expenditure, and how much fat you have on your body.

I found a study from 2005 that went back to analyze the data from the Minnesota Starvation Experiment (which I describe in the introduction of *Fast. Feast. Repeat.*). They found a maximum "fat loss" formula of (290+/-25) kJ/kgd. What the heck does that even mean?

Good news! I don't need to know what it means or how to do that math. Instead, I did a quick Google search using that formula and found a blog post where someone had performed some calculations using that formula, and they estimated that a 280-pound man with 37 percent body fat could possibly lose 6.4 pounds of fat per week at best, while a 180-pound man with 10 percent body fat has the potential to lose 1.1 pounds of fat per week. That's with zero food coming in at all, which isn't recommended, of course. We fast, FEAST, repeat.

I haven't verified that blog post math, and keep in mind

that it's all theoretical anyway. My point, though, is that nobody's losing thirty-two pounds of fat in two weeks. The body can't do that.

Why did I share all of that with you? For one very important reason: to succeed as an intermittent faster, you need to have realistic expectations.

Over the years, I've seen intermittent fasters who are having wonderful success—losing from one-half to one pound per week—*quit IF* and go on a crash diet, simply because they weren't losing weight as quickly as they expected. As with all crash diets, they may lose scale weight a lot more quickly than they were doing with IF, but it always comes back just as quickly. When the crash diet is over, we usually gain weight even faster than we lost it. We also usually end up losing significant lean tissue on a crash diet, so when we regain the lost weight, we are flabbier than we were before we began.

I've also seen other intermittent fasters who relax into the process and embrace their "slow" (yet actually *normal*) rate of loss of one-half to one pound per week.

Guess which person has made substantial progress one year later, and guess which one is "restarting" IF yet again?

I want you to avoid the "I must lose as much weight as I can, as fast as I can" trap.

To avoid that trap, there are several things you can do. Don't read those magazine headlines and compare your rate of loss to those outlandish and unrealistic claims. Don't be seduced by your friend's Facebook or Instagram posts about her weight-loss coaching program where you'll lose weight quickly (usually, you'll also need to buy special and expensive supplements or foods). Avoid news articles about new "miracle" weight-loss drugs.

After your FAST Start is over, you'll begin weighing daily and calculating your weekly average. You'll learn to ignore daily fluctuations, and only pay attention to your overall trend from week to week.

Most importantly, you'll be satisfied with a rate of loss of one-half to one pound per week. That may not sound sexy, and it certainly isn't making headlines on supermarket shelves, but it's reality . . . and every pound adds up over time.

DAILY INSPIRATION SPOTLIGHT:
Beth Anundi, Sublimity, Oregon
Intermittent Fasting Stories guest, episode 247

How long has she been an intermittent faster? *Between two and three years.*

If migraines are a part of your life, you may empathize with my intermittent fasting origin story because migraines were just a part of life for me from the time I started college in 1989. My migraines had started to truly interrupt my life on a grand scale by 2016, and by 2020, I was out of commission with a migraine for a minimum of two to six days every month. Because it had escalated to this degree, I had started physical therapy and massage alongside medication to try to combat them. When the doctor recommended I take a pill daily to keep them at bay, I knew it was time to think differently. Googling led me to Fast. Feast. Repeat. by Gin Stephens, and I started fasting that evening as I read her book. Honestly, I didn't think fasting would work to get rid of migraines, but I realized that if nothing else had helped, what was the harm in try-

ing this crazy thing of not eating for hours on end. I mean, really?!?! I love to eat, so I bought into the idea of Delay, Don't Deny *fairly heavily, and the first day at twenty hours fasted, I opened my feasting window with a trip to Dairy Queen for a chicken strip meal followed by a Blizzard. Yep, you read that right, and then I ate my dinner as well and closed my window within four hours. I stuck to the 20:4 pattern for several months and my migraines diminished to zero within five months . . . and I was losing weight! This was shocking, and when I noticed the weight loss, I tweaked my window over the course of the following year and tried all types of different patterns to see if I could lose more weight. Over the course of one year—to the day—I lost thirty-five pounds, ditched the migraines, and started sleeping better than I had in years. I am now able to easily rise in the early morning (my family can tell stories about what a horrific person I used to be in the morning); I no longer suffer from seasonal affective disorder; my allergies have dissipated significantly; the pain I couldn't explain in my lower back is gone; the unexplained pain between my shoulder blades is gone. My hearing is better because my allergies are pretty much gone, and one of my favorite non-scale victories to date is the fact that my skin no longer negatively reacts to the sun! The positive life-altering benefits I've experienced because of intermittent fasting mean I never had to take that daily migraine medication, and I haven't taken any migraine meds for months! I believe the benefits of resting from digestion have probably saved me from a host of health issues I may have seen as I entered my fifties, and I look forward to the future of a fasting lifestyle unlike any other lifestyle change I have ever embarked upon.*

24

ADVICE FROM BETH

The greatest keys to resting from digestion are to make sure you rest from digestion each and every day—don't stop fasting but instead alter it to fit your lifestyle so you can enjoy the benefits—and be sure to clean fast—eating is eating and fasting is fasting; if you have to ask if you can have it while fasted, the answer is likely nope—and be in a community with those who believe that fasting is fasting and eating is eating (the clean fast matters).

YOU HAVE ALL THE TOOLS YOU NEED TO SUCCEED. ENJOY YOUR DAY! YOU'VE GOT THIS.

HOW DID IT GO?
IT'S TIME TO REFLECT ON DAY 24.

TODAY (CHECK ALL THAT APPLY):

❏ I fasted clean (plain water, unflavored sparkling water, black unflavored coffee, plain tea)
❏ During the fast, I took time to reflect on the positive changes happening in my body
❏ Within my eating window, I ate until I was satisfied, and then I stopped
❏ I honored my "I've had enough" signals
❏ I stayed off the scale

FAST CHECK-IN

Rate the difficulty of today's fast on a scale from 1 to 10 (circle one):

1   2   3   4   5   6   7   8   9   **10**

(Today was easy! I sailed right through it.)   (Today was HARD! I struggled.)

During today's fast, I felt _____
_____
_____
_____
_____
_____

(*examples: exhilarated, hopeful, hungry, uncomfortable, bored, etc.*)

I used these strategies to manage my feelings today (check all that apply and add your own):

- ❏ I remembered my *why*
- ❏ I stayed busy
- ❏ I enjoyed a clean-fast-safe beverage
- ❏ I went on a walk
- ❏ I imagined my body tapping into my fat stores for fuel
- ❏ _____
  _____
- ❏ _____
  _____
- ❏ _____
  _____

EATING WINDOW CHECK-IN

Eating Window Length Goal: _____ hours
Actual Eating Window Length: _____ hours

How do I feel about today's eating window?

_____
_____
_____
_____
_____
_____
_____
_____

What went well? Was there anything that I struggled with during my eating window? _____

_____

_____

_____

_____

_____

_____

_____

_____

_____

TODAY'S NSVS, OR NON-SCALE VICTORIES

One of the most powerful things we can do is acknowledge our Non-Scale Victories (NSVs). These can be physical (*pain reduction, better energy, mental clarity, etc.*) or emotional (*freedom around food, confidence, etc.*).

What were today's NSVs? _____

_____

_____

_____

_____

_____

_____

_____

_____

_____

REFLECTIONS

Today, I listened to my body when I: _____

_____

_____

_____

_____

_____

_____

_____

Today's *AHA!* moment(s): _____

_____

_____

_____

Something that is on my mind: _____

_____

_____

_____

PREPARING FOR SUCCESS

Goal(s) and/or strategies for tomorrow: _____

_____

_____

_____

_____

DAY 25: *TWEAK IT TILL IT'S EASY—* NOW AND IN THE FUTURE

Today's Date: _____

PLANNING FOR A SUCCESSFUL DAY 25

Today, I am following

25

- ❑ The *Easy Does It* Approach (six-hour window, including a low-carb ease-in lunch *or* snack, plus a regular dinner)
- ❑ The *Steady Build* Approach (five-hour window, including snack, and dinner)
- ❑ The *Rip Off the Band-Aid* Approach (four-hour window, including snack, and dinner)

My personal goal(s) for today: _____

_____

_____

_____

_____

Daily Lesson from Gin: Tweak it till it's easy—now and in the future.

On day 8, I told you that our goal is to tweak it till it's easy, and when I did, you were just a week into your FAST Start. Now you're on day 25 and nearing the end—though the end of the FAST Start is more of a new beginning than an "end," when you think about it. It's the time when you'll take off the training wheels of the FAST Start and bike off into the future. Like a kid on a new bike, you might be wobbly at first, but eventually you'll be confident in your ability to keep riding. Okay, maybe that's corny, but I always love an analogy.

On day 29 and beyond, the structure of the FAST Start will be over, and you may wonder what to do next.

Never fear! You're equipped with a whole toolbox full of tools and strategies to ensure that you have long-term IF success. Everything you need to customize a long-term IF lifestyle that works for you and helps you meet your goals is explained in *Fast. Feast. Repeat.*

I want to remind you of some of the most immediate tools at your disposal as you continue to tweak it till it's easy over the coming weeks and months. I shared some of these on day 8, but some of these are new:

- **Focus on the boundary of your daily eating window rather than the length of your fast**—For me, a five-hour eating window was my overall weight-loss sweet spot, though yours might be slightly longer or shorter than mine. (The eating window chapter of *Fast. Feast. Repeat.* can help you decide.) While we often call a five-hour daily eating window approach 19:5, that can make some people think they are *required* to always fast for nineteen hours or they aren't doing it right. That couldn't be further from the truth. For me, rather than count the hours I spent fasting, it has always been so much easier to open my window whenever it feels right each day and then close it within five hours.

Here's how this might look in practice: Maybe my normal routine is to open my window at 2:00 p.m. and close it by 7:00 p.m.—five hours. The next day, I might be busy and not open until 3:00 p.m. That would mean I would close by 8:00 p.m.—five hours. It's super easy to count to five.

Here's where people get tripped up. If I close at 8:00 p.m., nineteen hours from then is 3:00 p.m. the next day. If I am doing 19:5, don't I have to wait nineteen hours to open? The answer is NO. Open whenever you want—as long as you stick to the five-hour eating window boundary. If you average five hours a day for your eating window, your fast will *average* nineteen hours a day. No need to stress about the exact numbers from day to day. Keep the boundary of your daily eating window and the fast will take care of itself over time. (Note: I no longer count my daily eating window hours, because I have been an intermittent faster for so long that it is simply what I do with no need to count hours—but as you're cementing your IF habit, counting your daily window hours is a great strategy. Otherwise, you may start to experience "window creep," where your window stretches longer and longer because you aren't paying attention. If you realize that is happening, simply tighten things back up again.)

- **Appreciate what is happening in your body during the daily fast**—Rather than thinking the fast is something you have to "get through" to reach your eating window, remember the power of the clean fast. Every day, you're experiencing increased autophagy and activating your body's fat-burning superpower. You don't want to give that up simply because your friends are drinking creamy lattes or having a snack. Honor your daily fast, recognize all the amazing things your body is doing, and delay. The minute I changed my focus from "getting through" each fast to appreciating each fast, it changed the whole experience.

- **Plan for eating window success**—As I already mentioned, it can be very helpful to have a plan for how you will open your eating window. That can prevent the experience of wandering around the kitchen eating anything you can find. Even now, if I don't have something satisfying on hand when I open my window, I might find myself making questionable eating choices.

- **Focus on foods that satisfy your body**—While you always get to eat what *you* want, some foods are going to be better choices than others. Our bodies are searching for nutrients, and whenever you can choose high-quality real foods over ultra-processed foods, your body is going to be more satisfied. I don't want you to think of foods as "good" or "bad" but instead think of foods as "satisfying" or "unsatisfying." As an example, if I opened my window with a bag of potato chips, I wouldn't be very satisfied. A huge loaded baked potato, however? I would feel extremely satisfied after eating that.

- **Play with your window timing**—It's fine to shift your daily eating window around. Not everyone has the same eating window sweet spot, and you'll never know what works best for you until you try some things that *don't* work. You always have permission to experiment. Maybe you're someone who does best with an early eating window. Maybe you do best with a midday window. Or perhaps you're like me—I feel my best with an eating window that closes a couple of hours before bedtime.

DAILY INSPIRATION SPOTLIGHT:
Sunshine, from Maine
Intermittent Fasting Stories guest, episode 133

How long has she been an intermittent faster? *Between two and three years.*

I started intermittent fasting in January of 2019 because my husband was diagnosed with diabetes. His nurse told him to read The Obesity Code *by Jason Fung. I bought him a copy, and he didn't read it. So, I read it. I'd heard about fasting from Michael Mosley's* The Fast Diet, *and I did that off and on, but it was so hard with the five hundred calories spaced throughout the day. Now I know that I kept spiking my insulin every time I ate a five-calorie pickle or drank coffee with vegan cream, so I never got into fat burning. I then listened to* Intermittent Fasting Stories, *which I listened to every time an episode came out. I would use these podcasts as motivation in the early stages when I was working through hunger. I bought* Delay, Don't Deny *on Audible and Kindle as well as* Fast. Feast. Repeat. *when that finally came out.* Fast.

25

Feast. Repeat. *is my favorite book ever! I lost forty pounds the first year and ten more pounds the second year. I have maintained the same weight for another year. After the first six months, the pain in my knees went away. I have so much more energy now than I did before fasting. I feel physically stronger and have more mental focus than before. Food tastes better. My relationship with food has improved, and I no longer measure food or eliminate certain foods. I am vegan for the animals and for the planet. I have been vegan for thirty years, and that will never change, but I no longer try to limit olive oil or measure my pasta (I threw out my pasta-measuring gadget). If I have a longer eating window than my body wanted, I just move on, and don't beat myself up like I used to when I'd overeat before fasting. Now, three years into intermittent fasting, I am less hungry than I used to be before fasting (because I am metabolically flexible and switch easily to fat burning). This power in my body has really improved my sense of self. Intermittent fasting has given me so much more self-confidence. I'm still working on how to eat during a rushed lunch with twelve-plus-hour nursing shifts. I'm not sure I'll ever figure this one out, but that's okay.*

ADVICE FROM SUNSHINE

I started fasting with a sixteen-hour eating window. I shrank that eating window slowly, by about half an hour a day until I had only an eight-hour eating window. Then I shortened it by an hour a week for a few weeks. Now I have anywhere from a thirty-minute window at work to a six-hour window on some days off. Go slowly. Figure out what works for your body and your life. Listen to your body and the podcasts!

**YOU HAVE ALL THE TOOLS YOU NEED TO SUCCEED.
ENJOY YOUR DAY! YOU'VE GOT THIS.**

25

HOW DID IT GO?

IT'S TIME TO REFLECT ON DAY 25.

TODAY (CHECK ALL THAT APPLY):

- ❏ I fasted clean (plain water, unflavored sparkling water, black unflavored coffee, plain tea)
- ❏ During the fast, I took time to reflect on the positive changes happening in my body
- ❏ Within my eating window, I ate until I was satisfied, and then I stopped
- ❏ I honored my "I've had enough" signals
- ❏ I stayed off the scale

FAST CHECK-IN

Rate the difficulty of today's fast on a scale from 1 to 10 (circle one):

1　2　3　4　5　6　7　8　9　**10**

(Today was easy! I sailed right through it.)　　(Today was HARD! I struggled.)

During today's fast, I felt _____
_____
_____
_____
_____
_____

(*examples: exhilarated, hopeful, hungry, uncomfortable, bored, etc.*)

I used these strategies to manage my feelings today (check all that apply and add your own):

- ❏ I remembered my *why*
- ❏ I stayed busy
- ❏ I enjoyed a clean-fast-safe beverage
- ❏ I went on a walk
- ❏ I imagined my body tapping into my fat stores for fuel
- ❏ _____
  _____
- ❏ _____
  _____
- ❏ _____
  _____

EATING WINDOW CHECK-IN

Eating Window Length Goal: _____ hours
Actual Eating Window Length: _____ hours

How do I feel about today's eating window?

_____
_____
_____
_____
_____
_____
_____
_____
_____
_____

What went well? Was there anything that I struggled with during my eating window? _____

_____

_____

_____

_____

_____

_____

_____

_____

_____

TODAY'S NSVS, OR NON-SCALE VICTORIES

One of the most powerful things we can do is acknowledge our Non-Scale Victories (NSVs). These can be physical (*pain reduction, better energy, mental clarity, etc.*) or emotional (*freedom around food, confidence, etc.*).

What were today's NSVs? _____

_____

_____

_____

_____

_____

_____

_____

_____

REFLECTIONS

Today, I listened to my body when I: _____

_____

_____

_____

_____

_____

_____

_____

Today's *AHA!* moment(s): _____

_____

_____

_____

Something that is on my mind: _____

_____

_____

_____

PREPARING FOR SUCCESS

Goal(s) and/or strategies for tomorrow: _____

_____

_____

_____

_____

DAY 26: DISCIPLINE *IS* REQUIRED: MASTERING THE "DELAY"

Today's Date: _____

PLANNING FOR A SUCCESSFUL DAY 26

Today, I am following

- ❏ The *Easy Does It* Approach (six-hour window, including a low-carb ease-in lunch *or* snack, plus a regular dinner)
- ❏ The *Steady Build* Approach (five-hour window, including snack, and dinner)
- ❏ The *Rip Off the Band-Aid* Approach (four-hour window, including snack, and dinner)

My personal goal(s) for today: _____

_____

_____

_____

_____

Daily Lesson from Gin: Discipline is required: mastering the "delay"

When I wrote my first intermittent fasting book in 2016, I gave it a title that represented my IF philosophy: "Delay, Don't Deny." It has become my mantra over the years, and thousands of IFers have agreed that those words represent how they want to live their lives.

Let's think about those words:

Delay, Don't Deny.

When I am fasting, I know that I've chosen to delay my eating until later in the day. That's all I have to do. Delay until later. I don't have to deny myself delicious and satisfying foods. When my window opens, I eat until I have had enough.

This lifestyle feels luxurious . . . once my window is open. But . . .

When I am fasting, I embrace the discipline of the delay.

Over time, I mastered the delay, and it allowed me to lose eighty pounds and keep it off. My daily IF schedule in maintenance allows for flexibility. Thankfully, I can be more flexible now within maintenance than I was when I was actively working to lose weight.

When I was in weight-loss mode, however, I needed consistency and discipline—daily. Occasionally, I could flex for a special occasion.

Key word: *occasionally.*

To get to the wonderfully flexible IF maintenance lifestyle I dreamed of (and am living today), I had to practice the daily "delay" consistently and for enough time to allow my body to burn fat. Being overly flexible would have gotten in the way of me reaching my weight-loss goals.

There will always be another holiday. Another vacation. Another summer. Another Christmas season. Another weekend.

As I already told you on day 7, Saturday is not a special occasion: it happens every week.

When your goal is weight loss, you need to have realistic

expectations about what is required. Fat loss doesn't happen without some sort of conscious decision, and you're going to need to focus on HOW it happens.

We say: delay, don't deny. But what if you struggle with the delay? You keep finding reasons to open early. "Today, I'm going to eat early. Tomorrow I'll fast." Only tomorrow, there's another reason you can't (or don't want to) delay.

For IF to be a successful weight-loss strategy, you MUST nail the "delay."

Want to lose weight? You get to choose. You can Delay OR you can Deny. Typical diets you did before? They are the "deny." Did you enjoy those diets? Did they work long term? Probably not, or you wouldn't be here.

IF can be freedom from the "deny," but only if you master the "delay."

You deserve to feel good in your own body. You DESERVE to delay.

Commit to YOURSELF.

So! What will YOU commit to as you approach the end of your FAST Start? When the novelty of IF wears off, how will you find the discipline you need to master the daily "delay"?

DAILY INSPIRATION SPOTLIGHT:
Star McEuen, Pima, Arizona
Intermittent Fasting Stories guest, episode 79

How long has she been an intermittent faster? *Between three and four years.* .

Most of my life, I was focused on my weight and wanted to be "skinny and/or fit." I basically tried every "diet" out there to lose weight, did all the at-home workouts, went to the gym, hired nutritionists, and they all led to the same places: failure, disappointment, and defeat. I hit thirty-five years old, and no matter what I did to lose weight before, nothing was working this time, and the weight just piled on. In May of 2019, I weighed in at 210 pounds. I was at the darkest point in my life. I was depressed, my health was deteriorating, I was tired, and I felt out of options. Then I found intermittent fasting in August of 2019, when my high school best friend shared that she had been intermittent fasting, and she recommended I try it. I read Delay, Don't Deny *and started with the clean fast and a 19:5-ish protocol, and by February of 2020, I had reached my first goal weight of 140 pounds. By August of 2020 (one year of fasting), I had lost a total of 81 pounds. My goal now is to get to twenty hours fasted most days, with a one- to four-hour eating window, with the occasional shorter fast and longer eating window, depending on my day. Fasting has taught me to be mindful of everything that goes into my body and to eat for nutrition and purpose. It has also taught me to think nutrients, NOT calories. I am no longer a prisoner to food. Food is not the enemy—too much circulating insulin is the problem. Fasting helps us regulate our hormones and helps us learn how to trust ourselves around food again. Fasting truly is the health plan with the side effect of weight loss, and I believe almost everyone should be an intermittent faster for the health benefits alone!*

26

ADVICE FROM STAR

To remember why *we fast, read the introduction and* chapters 1 and 2 of *Fast. Feast. Repeat. Never forget that we are looking for flexibility and sustainability.*

**YOU HAVE ALL THE TOOLS YOU NEED TO SUCCEED.
ENJOY YOUR DAY! YOU'VE GOT THIS.**

HOW DID IT GO?
IT'S TIME TO REFLECT ON DAY 26.

TODAY (CHECK ALL THAT APPLY):

- ❏ I fasted clean (plain water, unflavored sparkling water, black unflavored coffee, plain tea)
- ❏ During the fast, I took time to reflect on the positive changes happening in my body
- ❏ Within my eating window, I ate until I was satisfied, and then I stopped
- ❏ I honored my "I've had enough" signals
- ❏ I stayed off the scale

FAST CHECK-IN

Rate the difficulty of today's fast on a scale from 1 to 10 (circle one):

1 2 3 4 5 6 7 8 9 **10**

(Today was easy! I sailed right through it.)   (Today was HARD! I struggled.)

During today's fast, I felt _____
_____
_____
_____
_____
_____

(*examples: exhilarated, hopeful, hungry, uncomfortable, bored, etc.*)

I used these strategies to manage my feelings today (check all that apply and add your own):

- ❏ I remembered my *why*
- ❏ I stayed busy
- ❏ I enjoyed a clean-fast-safe beverage
- ❏ I went on a walk
- ❏ I imagined my body tapping into my fat stores for fuel
- ❏ _____
  _____
- ❏ _____
  _____
- ❏ _____
  _____

EATING WINDOW CHECK-IN

Eating Window Length Goal: _____ hours
Actual Eating Window Length: _____ hours

How do I feel about today's eating window?

_____
_____
_____
_____
_____
_____
_____
_____
_____

What went well? Was there anything that I struggled with during my eating window? _____

_____

_____

_____

_____

_____

_____

_____

_____

_____

_____

TODAY'S NSVS, OR NON-SCALE VICTORIES

One of the most powerful things we can do is acknowledge our Non-Scale Victories (NSVs). These can be physical (*pain reduction, better energy, mental clarity, etc.*) or emotional (*freedom around food, confidence, etc.*).

What were today's NSVs? _____

_____

_____

_____

_____

_____

_____

_____

_____

_____

REFLECTIONS

Today, I listened to my body when I: _____

_____

_____

_____

_____

_____

_____

Today's *AHA!* moment(s): _____

_____

_____

_____

Something that is on my mind: _____

_____

_____

_____

PREPARING FOR SUCCESS

Goal(s) and/or strategies for tomorrow: _____

_____

_____

_____

_____

DAY 27: HOW WILL YOU KNOW IF *IF* IS "WORKING"? REDEFINE *WORKING*

Today's Date: _____

PLANNING FOR A SUCCESSFUL DAY 27

Today, I am following

- ❏ The *Easy Does It* Approach (six-hour window, including a low-carb ease-in lunch *or* snack, plus a regular dinner)
- ❏ The *Steady Build* Approach (five-hour window, including snack, and dinner)
- ❏ The *Rip Off the Band-Aid* Approach (four-hour window, including snack, and dinner)

My personal goal(s) for today: _____

_____

_____

_____

_____

Daily Lesson from Gin: How will you know if IF is "working"? Redefine *working*.

"IF isn't working for me, Gin."

I have heard that statement so many times over the years. A new intermittent faster becomes discouraged because they get it in their heads that IF isn't "working."

I usually ask, "What do you mean by that?"

Ninety-nine times out of a hundred, the answer has something to do with lack of perceived weight loss.

As you get to the end of your FAST Start, you may remember that on day 29, I recommend that you once again weigh in, take measurements, and take progress photos. But you should also remember what I told you from the beginning: the FAST Start is *not* the time to expect weight loss.

It's very likely that your weight won't be down (and it might even be *up* slightly), your measurements won't have changed, and your progress photos won't show a noticeable difference.

That's when you start to question whether IF will "work" for you.

When you think IF isn't "working," that's when you're more likely to quit. But we're here to make sure that your IF lifestyle *sticks*. Being very clear about whether IF is "working" is an important part of the process.

I want to take you back to the beginning, when you defined your *why*. I asked you to consider this list, checking off anything that you wanted to include and adding your own:

- ❑ I want to lose weight and keep it off
- ❑ I want to feel good in my body
- ❑ I want to fit into clothes that make me feel wonderful when I wear them
- ❑ I want to get off medications
- ❑ I want to lower my A1C
- ❑ I want to change my entire health trajectory, so I age well and live a vibrant life
- ❑ I want to avoid diseases that are often linked to aging

❏ I want to be pain-free

❏ I want to have more physical endurance

❏ I want to maintain my muscle mass and become even stronger than I am now

❏ I want to enjoy foods again

❏ I want to cure my diet brain forever so I can stop trying to find yet another diet

❏ I want to be there for my family—my partner/spouse/ kids/grandkids—and for everyone I care about

❏ _____

_____

❏ _____

_____

❏ _____

_____

❏ _____

_____

❏ _____

_____

Which of those did you choose back then? Now that you are approaching the end of your FAST Start, would you choose differently today?

No matter what your answers to those two questions are, I think we can agree on this:

- If you never lose a pound, but you get off all medications, is IF "working"?

- If you never lose an inch, but your A1C normalizes, is IF "working"?

- If your clothes fit the same way in a year, but you're pain-free, is IF "working"?

The answer to each one of those questions, of course, is a resounding *YES*.

As you continue to live your intermittent fasting lifestyle after the FAST Start is over and throughout the first year, it's important to always keep your eyes on your *why* and to also recognize positive changes that are occurring along the way.

If you're experiencing powerful non-scale victories and feeling better, IF is working. If you're defeating decades of diet brain, IF is working!

Be confident with this thought: if you discover that weight loss is elusive or slower than you hoped for over the coming months, you'll be equipped with many powerful tools in your toolbox . . . *Fast. Feast. Repeat.* is *full of* tools. In our online support community, we help people apply those tools every day.

But always know this: no matter what your weight is doing, IF never stops "working." It is doing powerful things in your body.

DAILY INSPIRATION SPOTLIGHT:
Marie Todd, Moody, Alabama
Intermittent Fasting Stories guest, episode 88

How long has she been an intermittent faster? *Between four and five years.*

During my Intermittent Fasting Stories *episode, I often used the phrase* for me *because I truly believe the IF journey is a personal one. Just like no prescriptive food list or single fasting protocol is perfect for everyone—there is an answer for everyone. It may take time to get the right mindset and discover the protocol that works best for you. Then it may change. And change again. Because life changes, and you change. At the time of the February 2020 interview, I had lost about forty-two pounds and felt the absolute best of my life. My focus was not on the scale number but the true freedom I had found with fasting as a never-dieting-again lifestyle. Soon after, as many others experienced in March 2020, life changed dramatically for me. I continued fasting daily, but faced grief, stress, anxiety, and work changes. I did gain some weight during this period. But here's the good news: I reread* Fast. Feast. Repeat. *and my answers were there. I renewed my mindset. I rebooted with a different fasting protocol (the Steady Build Approach). I lost the weight I had gained. I'm not yet the perfect size or weight, but I am also not a miserable forever-dieter. I am a forever-free intermittent faster with hope and the tools to be successful.*

27

ADVICE FROM MARIE

My advice to a new intermittent faster or someone restarting is to DECIDE. Decide that you will learn, and try, and succeed, and slip, and persevere, and tweak, and keep deciding that this is your lifestyle. Forever. There is a lot of confusing fasting information online, but I trust the scientific research about the biology of why IF works, and the real-life experiences that Gin has presented in Fast. Feast. Repeat. *I mention this book not as an homage to her but because I*

> *believe that she compiled the absolute best resource available. Every time I pick up this guidebook, I learn something, gain greater understanding about myself, and discover the next steps in* my journey.

**YOU HAVE ALL THE TOOLS YOU NEED TO SUCCEED.
ENJOY YOUR DAY! YOU'VE GOT THIS.**

HOW DID IT GO?
IT'S TIME TO REFLECT ON DAY 27.

TODAY (CHECK ALL THAT APPLY):

❏ I fasted clean (plain water, unflavored sparkling water, black unflavored coffee, plain tea)
❏ During the fast, I took time to reflect on the positive changes happening in my body
❏ Within my eating window, I ate until I was satisfied, and then I stopped
❏ I honored my "I've had enough" signals
❏ I stayed off the scale

FAST CHECK-IN

Rate the difficulty of today's fast on a scale from 1 to 10 (circle one):

1 2 3 4 5 6 7 8 9 **10**

(Today was easy! I sailed right through it.)   (Today was HARD! I struggled.)

During today's fast, I felt _____
_____
_____
_____
_____
_____

(*examples: exhilarated, hopeful, hungry, uncomfortable, bored, etc.*)

I used these strategies to manage my feelings today (check all that apply and add your own):

- ❏ I remembered my *why*
- ❏ I stayed busy
- ❏ I enjoyed a clean-fast-safe beverage
- ❏ I went on a walk
- ❏ I imagined my body tapping into my fat stores for fuel
- ❏ _____
  _____
- ❏ _____
  _____
- ❏ _____
  _____

EATING WINDOW CHECK-IN

Eating Window Length Goal: _____ hours
Actual Eating Window Length: _____ hours

How do I feel about today's eating window?

_____
_____
_____
_____
_____
_____
_____
_____
_____

What went well? Was there anything that I struggled with during my eating window? _____

_____

_____

_____

_____

_____

_____

_____

_____

_____

TODAY'S NSVS, OR NON-SCALE VICTORIES

One of the most powerful things we can do is acknowledge our Non-Scale Victories (NSVs). These can be physical (*pain reduction, better energy, mental clarity, etc.*) or emotional (*freedom around food, confidence, etc.*).

What were today's NSVs? _____

_____

_____

_____

_____

_____

_____

_____

_____

REFLECTIONS

Today, I listened to my body when I: _____

_____

_____

_____

_____

_____

_____

Today's *AHA!* moment(s): _____

_____

_____

_____

Something that is on my mind: _____

_____

_____

_____

PREPARING FOR SUCCESS

Goal(s) and/or strategies for tomorrow: _____

_____

_____

_____

_____

DAY 28: PLANNING FOR SUCCESS: COMMIT TO TWELVE MONTHS, NO MATTER WHAT HAPPENS

Today's Date: _____

PLANNING FOR A SUCCESSFUL DAY 28

Today, I am following

❏ The *Easy Does It* Approach (six-hour window, including a low-carb ease-in lunch *or* snack, plus a regular dinner)
❏ The *Steady Build* Approach (five-hour window, including snack, and dinner)
❏ The *Rip Off the Band-Aid* Approach (four-hour window, including snack, and dinner)

My personal goal(s) for today: _____

_____

_____

_____

_____

28

Daily Lesson from Gin: Planning for success: commit to twelve months, no matter what happens.

Okay, so it's not really "no matter what happens" . . . there are a couple of scenarios that would mean you actually should stop fasting: please stop fasting if you get pregnant (fasting is not recommended while you're growing a new human, and that also includes the time when you're breastfeeding) or if your doctor gives you a medical reason why you need to set fasting aside for a time. Other than those two instances, though, committing to twelve months is the best thing you can do for yourself.

And here's some good news: YOU ARE ALREADY ONE-TWELFTH OF THE WAY through your first year. If that's not something to celebrate, I don't know what is.

Twelve months after you began IF, you'll be ready to celebrate your first fast-iversary. And that is a big deal! When a member of our online community celebrates his or her first (or second, or third . . .) fast-iversary, we all celebrate. The more years you spend as an IFer, the more it simply becomes who you are.

I am an intermittent faster.

It's part of my identity now. I don't have to stress about it or think about it. I don't have to plan for it. It's simply what I *do*.

It didn't happen overnight. It didn't happen in the first month, as a matter of fact. I wish I could pinpoint the moment when it happened. I can't.

But it eventually does happen for everyone . . . even YOU.

As long as you don't stop.

The best recipe for intermittent fasting success is to get up every day and do it again.

Some days, you'll have shorter fasts and longer windows. Some days, fasting will be hard. Some days, you'll push through the hard, and other days you won't. Eventually, you'll know when your body needs a day or two with more food and you will no longer stress about it.

Tomorrow, you'll get back on the scale (only if you choose to—it isn't required) and you'll take new progress photos (wearing the same outfit you wore on day 0).

And when you do, remember what I said:

Commit to twelve months, no matter what happens.

Don't forget that the 28-Day FAST Start was not the time to expect weight loss or body changes. You may even find that your weight is *UP* and your clothes are tighter.

While that won't feel awesome, promise me (and more importantly, promise *yourself*) that you aren't going to allow that to derail you or shake your confidence.

I promise—you are not the one person that IF won't work for.

28

But it takes time.

During the FAST Start, your body has been learning how to do something new. When you started, your body wasn't skilled at tapping into fat stores for fuel (and it's possible that your body still hasn't flipped that metabolic switch . . . but it *will*).

Because your body has had to learn how to tap into your fat stores, it's extremely likely that you've had very little fat loss by this point. Also, during the time when your body wasn't yet metabolically flexible, you may have found that you were hungrier than usual. This happens when your body isn't well fueled during the fast. When your window opened, you got the signal to eat and eat—so you may have had some overeating for a time.

Put these factors together, and that's why some people see a little weight gain during the FAST Start.

This does NOT mean IF won't "work" for you.

Remember that on day 27, we redefined what it means for IF to "work" for you. Always remember that it never *stops* working.

So, no matter what happens on day 29 when it comes to your weight or your progress photos, commit to the next eleven months, no matter what.

Before you know it, we'll be celebrating YOUR fast-iversary.

DAILY INSPIRATION SPOTLIGHT:
Heather Stuart, New Zealand
Intermittent Fasting Stories guest, episode 97

How long has she been an intermittent faster? *Between three and four years.*

Four years ago, I was fifty-eight, 1.5 meters tall (4' 11"), and 90.6 kilograms (199.7 pounds) . . . uncomfortable, unconfident, and I did not want to be the mother of the groom in this shape, again. A friend mentioned fasting, and I googled. After a year, I was around 60 kilograms (132 pounds)! Intermittent fasting had changed my life. It was about this time Gin interviewed me. I was so nervous, but really wished to share my story, and it was such an honor to speak to my mentor. Today, I'm averaging around 58 kilograms (127 pounds). I thought I'd like to be 55 kilo-

grams (121 pounds), but why? I like the size of the clothes I wear now (my favorite trousers don't even come in a smaller size!), and I feel better than I have in decades. I have many NSVs, including many health victories. IF has been life-changing for me in so many ways. My confidence has improved, I now participate rather than spectate, and I love trying new activities. Buying clothes is fun again! I know I have added years to my life. People say, "You're so disciplined." But honestly, it feels so natural.

ADVICE FROM HEATHER

We are all so different from each other, so don't expect your journey to be the same as someone else's; your body will decide what healing to focus on first. I didn't get on the scales for the first month as Gin recommends, and it was so worth it.

**YOU HAVE ALL THE TOOLS YOU NEED TO SUCCEED.
ENJOY YOUR DAY! YOU'VE GOT THIS.**

28

HOW DID IT GO?
IT'S TIME TO REFLECT ON DAY 28.

TODAY (CHECK ALL THAT APPLY):

- ❏ I fasted clean (plain water, unflavored sparkling water, black unflavored coffee, plain tea)
- ❏ During the fast, I took time to reflect on the positive changes happening in my body
- ❏ Within my eating window, I ate until I was satisfied, and then I stopped
- ❏ I honored my "I've had enough" signals
- ❏ I stayed off the scale

FAST CHECK-IN

Rate the difficulty of today's fast on a scale from 1 to 10 (circle one):

1　2　3　4　5　6　7　8　9　**10**

(Today was easy! I sailed right through it.)　　　(Today was HARD! I struggled.)

During today's fast, I felt _____

_____

_____

_____

_____

_____

(*examples: exhilarated, hopeful, hungry, uncomfortable, bored, etc.*)

I used these strategies to manage my feelings today (check all that apply and add your own):

- ❏ I remembered my *why*
- ❏ I stayed busy
- ❏ I enjoyed a clean-fast-safe beverage
- ❏ I went on a walk
- ❏ I imagined my body tapping into my fat stores for fuel
- ❏ _____
  _____
- ❏ _____
  _____
- ❏ _____
  _____

EATING WINDOW CHECK-IN

Eating Window Length Goal: _____ hours
Actual Eating Window Length: _____ hours

How do I feel about today's eating window?

_____
_____
_____
_____
_____
_____
_____
_____
_____

What went well? Was there anything that I struggled with during my eating window? _____

_____

_____

_____

_____

_____

_____

_____

_____

_____

TODAY'S NSVS, OR NON-SCALE VICTORIES

One of the most powerful things we can do is acknowledge our Non-Scale Victories (NSVs). These can be physical (*pain reduction, better energy, mental clarity, etc.*) or emotional (*freedom around food, confidence, etc.*).

What were today's NSVs? _____

_____

_____

_____

_____

_____

_____

_____

REFLECTIONS

Today, I listened to my body when I: _____

_____

_____

_____

_____

_____

_____

_____

Today's *AHA!* moment(s): _____

_____

_____

_____

Something that is on my mind: _____

_____

_____

_____

PREPARING FOR SUCCESS

Goal(s) and/or strategies for tomorrow: _____

_____

_____

_____

_____

DAY 29: YOU DID IT! TAKING STOCK OF YOUR FAST START

After following the FAST Start for twenty-eight days, it's time to repeat your measurements and photos:

DAY 29 . . . FAST START COMPLETED!

Date: _____

Current weight: _____

Measurements: _____

    Bust or chest: _____

    Waist: _____

    Hips: _____

    Right thigh: _____

    Left thigh: _____

Put on the same outfit that you wore on day 0 and take photos from the same exact angles that you did before: front, side, and back. Try to re-create the photos as closely as possible. Compare the photos from day 0 to the ones you took on day 29.

Here is something that is *really important* that I have already mentioned throughout your FAST Start: the FAST Start is not the time to expect weight loss. You may not have lost a single pound. Your measurements may not have changed at all. Your photos may look exactly the same. Or your weight/measurements might be *up*. Your clothes might be *tighter*.

Deep breath. That is okay. It's *all* okay. The 28-Day FAST Start is *not* the weight-loss phase . . . it's the adjustment phase. Now that your body has had twenty-eight days to adjust to IF, you are ready to begin weighing daily. You will begin taking biweekly measurements and progress photos now. The FAST Start is over, and *now* is the time to expect slow-yet-steady progress. Chapter 18 of *Fast. Feast. Repeat.*, "Scale-Schmale: The Ultimate Guide to Tracking Your Progress," explains all the ways you should track your progress going forward, so your homework is to go ahead and read that chapter if you haven't read it recently.

CONGRATULATIONS to you! You're on your way.

Before you do anything else, I want you to take some time to write a letter to yourself. This letter is for you in eleven months, on your first fast-iversary.

In this letter, visualize *you*, eleven months into the future. How will your life be different eleven months from now, on your first fast-iversary? Did you have any struggles? How did you overcome them? What have been your greatest victories? How's your health?

Dream big! You're designing your future here.

29

Dear ME:

Today is _____*, and it's my first fast-iversary. I did it! I didn't quit.* _____

_____

_____

_____

_____

_____

_____
_____
_____
_____
_____
_____
_____
_____
_____
_____
_____
_____
_____
_____
_____
_____
_____

29

With lots of love and gratitude. Thank you for not quitting.

Sincerely,

_____

NEXT STEPS: WEEKS 5 AND BEYOND ... IF FOR L*IF*E ... TRUST THE PROCESS

Now that you've finished the FAST Start, I have some next steps for you.

1. **Read chapter 11 of *Fast. Feast. Repeat.*, "Tweak it Till It's Easy."** I have included a brief excerpt of that chapter in this book (following this section) to get you started, but the complete chapter has more than I included here.

2. **Read chapter 18 of *Fast. Feast. Repeat.*, "Scale-Schmale: The Ultimate Guide to Tracking Your Progress."** It's essential that you have a plan for tracking your progress over time. As I mentioned on day 24, realistic expectations make a powerful difference. You aren't going to lose thirty pounds in sixty days, but the "Scale-Schmale" chapter explains how to know for sure that you are making progress. And if you aren't making progress, you'll know. The good news is that

Fast. Feast. Repeat. has all the tools you'll need to change things up so you meet your long-term goals.

3. **Keep doing what you are doing.** The best way to have long-term success? Don't stop. Fast, feast, and repeat. I love to say, "The magic is in the clean fast," but the *real* magic is in the "repeat."

4. **Trust the process.** What does that mean? Does it mean that you keep doing what you are doing even if you aren't making progress? Yes, but also NO. I do want you to keep doing what you are doing, meaning keep fasting clean. But the *process* I want you to *trust* is the process of tweaking it till it's easy. *Tweaking* implies that you may need to change things up over time. *That*, my friend, is *the process*. Knowing what to tweak and when. All the tools you need are right there in *Fast. Feast. Repeat.*

5. **Start at the beginning of *Fast. Feast. Repeat.* and read it straight through.** I am a teacher, and I understand the power of repetition. When you hear something for the first time, you may not even have enough experience to know what you're reading. Now, though, you are an intermittent faster with twenty-eight days behind you. You'll understand what you're reading a lot more today than you would have on day 1, because of everything you've already experienced.

6. **You are forbidden to use the words *starting over*.** I'm not kidding. You are not allowed to "start over," because you aren't going to quit. I said that in my most loving teacher voice, and I meant it. Maybe you'll have a holiday season or a vacation and you'll be loosey-goosey with your fasting and feasting, but never forget

that you didn't "stop," and you don't need to "start over."

7. **Come back to *Fast. Feast. Repeat.* periodically.** As I mentioned already, I believe in the power of repetition. Every time you read and reread, you'll understand something better than you did the last time, and you'll be even more confident in the intermittent fasting lifestyle. Already read the paperback? Maybe it's time to get the audiobook and let me read it to you. You'll hear things differently from when you read them.

Just in case you haven't followed my instructions (and you don't yet have a copy of *Fast. Feast. Repeat.*), I am including an excerpt from chapter 11 here, which is the chapter following the FAST Start chapter.

That being said: you absolutely need a copy of *Fast. Feast. Repeat.* going forward, because it has everything you need along the way as you transition from the FAST Start to IF for L*IF*E.

EXCERPT FROM CHAPTER 11 OF *FAST. FEAST. REPEAT.*

You made it! You have finished the FAST Start, and now you are ready to take charge of your own IF plan going forward! Ready, set, go!

Um. What now? WHAT DO I DO, GIN???

Great question! You may be used to flipping through the pages of any new diet book looking for the exact "diet" or "meal plan" that the author has laid out for you. You know, the weekly schedule that everyone needs to follow to find success. Usually, there are phases and recipes and grocery lists and step-by-step guidelines for every part of the process. Well, you won't find that here.

IF is not a diet and there is no one-size-fits-all plan. This may be scary, because you are used to someone else telling you exactly what to do. I am not going to do that for you. As I told you in the beginning pages of this book, *you* are in charge. Why? Because I want *you* to feel empowered to find the right IF routine that works for you. It won't look exactly like mine.

It comes down to this:

Intermittent fasting is very personal.

I am sure you are wondering: How long do you need to fast every day for best results? What foods will make you feel best? What will the lifestyle look like for *you* long term? These are all excellent questions!

There's a pretty common phenomenon in any weight-loss support group. Any time someone shares about their success, others always ask: *What did you eat? When did you eat it? Tell us exactly what you did!*

It's natural for us to think that there is a magical answer out there that is the same for everyone. After all, isn't that what every diet plan has *always* told us? Do x, y, and z, exactly like this, and you'll lose weight.

How did that work for you? It probably *didn't* work for you long term, in fact, or you wouldn't be here.

Remember these three simple words: FAST. FEAST. REPEAT.

Your intermittent fasting lifestyle will have periods of fasting, periods of feasting, and you will repeat, alternating fasting with feasting. That's it.

And also remember this: ONE SIZE DOES NOT FIT ALL!

This brings up a very important point, and the point of this chapter. We have one more saying in our community that is the key to your personal success:

Tweak it till it's easy.

That saying is meant to empower you. After the 28-Day FAST Start, your body is getting into the fasting groove. While I did give you a few schedules to choose from and follow as your body adjusted to intermittent fasting and fat burning, your next step is to experiment with the various tools from the fasting toolbox.

We are taking off the training wheels, and you are ready to ride the bike! And, like a kid riding for the first time, you may worry that you can't do it without me holding on to the back of the bike.

You can! I promise you can.

Imagine me running along beside you, encouraging you every step of the way as you begin experimenting with the tools from your IF toolbox. You might fall down, but you'll dust yourself off and get right back on the bike!

As you experiment, remember that other than the clean fast (which is NOT optional, I promise), don't try to fit what you are doing into someone else's recommendations of how and when to fast (or even what you should be eating). Listen to how you feel over time and live your life as a study of one. The one that you are studying is *you*, and no one else knows what feels right to you better than, well, *you*.

The intermittent fasting lifestyle that makes *me* feel best is not necessarily the one that will make *you* feel best. And guess what else? The fasting pattern that feels effortless to you today may not feel effortless to you next month. You may need to go back to the toolbox, pick a new strategy, and try a different fasting pattern for a while. Don't be afraid to mix and match!

Tweak it till it's easy!

Want more? *Fast. Feast. Repeat.* has all the tools you need for success beyond the FAST Start . . . so your IF lifestyle sticks.

If you're looking for a support community, visit ginstephens.com/community to join us. I love nothing more than watching IFers succeed and cheer one another on. I'm there, as well.

And when you are ready to take things up a notch, you're ready for my follow-up book *Clean(ish): Eat (Mostly) Clean, Live (Mainly) Clean, and Unlock Your Body's Natural Ability to Self-Clean.*

ACKNOWLEDGMENTS

I would like to take a moment to express gratitude for every person who has been a part of both my intermittent fasting journey and my publishing path as an author and a podcaster. All of you who have been a part of my IF support communities, the amazing podcast guests I've been privileged to interview over the years, the support staff behind the scenes at St. Martin's Press and Macmillan, and everyone on my podcast production teams. I would not be here without all of you. If you're reading this and wondering, "Does Gin mean me?" the answer is yes. YOU. I couldn't have done it without you.

Elizabeth, Jaidree and Celeste, Sheri and Roxi—especially you. Thank you. And, to my family—thank you for always allowing me to be myself, even when it means I'm excitedly talking to strangers in line at the grocery store.

INDEX

ABOUT THE AUTHOR

GIN STEPHENS, the *New York Times* bestselling author of *Fast. Feast. Repeat.*, *Clean(ish)*, and *Delay, Don't Deny*, has lived the intermittent fasting lifestyle since 2014. Since then, she's maintained a weight loss of more than eighty pounds, launched an IF support website, and hosts two top-ranked podcasts: *Intermittent Fasting Stories* and *Fast. Feast. Repeat. Intermittent Fasting for Life*. She lives in Surfside Beach, South Carolina.

Visit the author at www.ginstephens.com.

Read more by *New York Times* bestselling author
GIN STEPHENS!

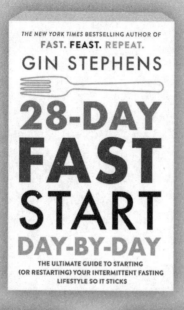

THE NEW YORK TIMES BESTSELLING AUTHOR OF
FAST. FEAST. REPEAT.
GIN STEPHENS
28-DAY
FAST
START
DAY-BY-DAY
**THE ULTIMATE GUIDE TO STARTING
(OR RESTARTING) YOUR INTERMITTENT FASTING
LIFESTYLE SO IT STICKS**

THE *NEW YORK TIMES* BESTSELLING AUTHOR OF
FAST. FEAST. REPEAT.
GIN STEPHENS
CLEAN(ISH)
FOREWORD BY
DR. TIM SPECTOR,
AUTHOR OF
SPOON FED

**EAT (MOSTLY) CLEAN, LIVE (MAINLY) CLEAN,
AND UNLOCK YOUR BODY'S NATURAL
ABILITY TO SELF-CLEAN**

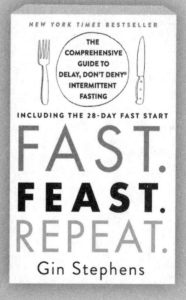

NEW YORK TIMES BESTSELLER
THE
COMPREHENSIVE
GUIDE TO
DELAY, DON'T DENY®
INTERMITTENT
FASTING
INCLUDING THE 28-DAY FAST START
FAST.
FEAST.
REPEAT.
Gin Stephens

ST. MARTIN'S GRIFFIN